CANCER
VERSUS
THE
HUMAN
SPIRIT

The Story of My Battle with Cancer
and How I Deal with the Disease

WILLIAM H. FLICK

authorHOUSE®

AuthorHouse™
1663 Liberty Drive
Bloomington, IN 47403
www.authorhouse.com
Phone: 1 (800) 839-8640

Published by AuthorHouse 10/26/2017

ISBN: 978-1-5462-1294-2 (sc)
ISBN: 978-1-5462-1293-5 (e)

Library of Congress Control Number: 2017915851

Print information available on the last page.

Any people depicted in stock imagery provided by Thinkstock are models,
and such images are being used for illustrative purposes only.
Certain stock imagery © Thinkstock.

This book is printed on acid-free paper.

CONTENTS

FOREWORD

This is the story of my battle with cancer. It is a story of the strength of the Human Spirit and the Holy Spirit. This book will hopefully be read by people afflicted with Cancer or those of you who know someone that is. I am not looking for pity or sympathy. I hope that if you are reading this, you or your loved ones may find a way to help deal with this terrible disease. If you are not really a big reader, do not worry it is a quick read. It is meant to be food for thought so to say. I am not going to make any stupid statements like, "I don't want to offend anyone", or such as that. These days you cannot help but offend someone. I will say, I do not mean to hurt anyone with what I have written here. At times my words may seem cold and harsh to some but this is a disease is not something to be taken light heartedly. It must be fought with cold harsh determination in order to survive. There is no room for light heartedness. I am trying to portray how much the human body and spirit can take and still go on. It is a story of endurance and tenacity of the spirit.

My statements are meant to reflect how I am seeing God, ourselves and life in relationship to this disease. Some of these words may apply to you personally and some are just referring to the behavior of people in general. I ask that you approach this book with an open mind looking for help and maybe a few answers. I am basically just a normal every day human being just like most of you. I grew up and do still live in a middle class home in Northeast Indiana. I tell you this because I want you to understand there is nothing special about me. I have no special skills or education that make me even remotely qualified to even think about writing a book. I have not studied under the "Dali Lama" or some far eastern mystic that makes me any stronger or smarter than you. I possess no supernatural techniques or anything of that nature. I am just a guy. I am actually not even a writer but after enough people told me I needed to write book and tell my story, I finally decided I had to do it.

I am writing this book to show people there is hope for people who have been afflicted with this terrible disease we call Cancer. I have discovered that after people hear my story, it somehow makes them feel better. Somehow it makes their problems seem a little smaller I guess. Everyone tells me I am some kind of miracle guy or something for having survived this ordeal.....but I think not. I give credit to God and the people in the Medical Community who I know at this point, he guided. After you finish reading, you will understand there HAD to be what is commonly referred to as "Divine Intervention" by God on my behalf or I would not be alive. You will start to notice how much of what most would call "Coincidence" or "Luck" has occurred and seems to be an ongoing part of my life. I do not believe in coincidence or luck. I would also like to thank all of the Doctors and Nurses whose skills, knowledge and expertise have been a part of my healing and my continued life. And even though you may have heard stories to the contrary, almost every bit of my health care has been done through the Veteran's Administration Health Care System. My hat goes off to them. They are extremely overworked, underpaid and overloaded with patients. They struggle with trying to do the very best they can in a system that is bogged down with bureaucracy and too damn many regulations. They work hard to give our nation's veterans health care. They have my deepest gratitude.

I write this hoping that people will understand the sheer will of the Human Spirit and its ability to survive when pushed to the extreme. Our minds are able to make us do amazing things when we want something bad enough. As I have told my children their whole lives, "You Gotta Wanna". I firmly believe that there are spiritual and mental components to healing that are as powerful as medicine if not even more so. I am hoping that after reading this, it may change your perspective and help you see and deal with your illness in a different way. A way that makes you understand that your will power and prayer can become and enormous part of your getting better. Also, I will apologize ahead of time as I am finding that writing a book is no small task. I should also mention that if you are weak of stomach, this book may not be for you. I am very graphic to try and get people to understand the pain and suffering people who have this terrible disease are experiencing. Telling the detail and length of my medical history in an attempt to help you understand that there are others who are overcoming and making life better through the power of prayer, sheer will and downright personal fortitude. Against all odds, I am still surviving. As I like to say, "By the Grace of God, there Go I".

Our desire to live is inherent in us genetically. It is powerful when we can find our way to see outside our own immediate circumstances. It also seems that the desire to survive is stronger in some than in others. If you have a loved one with Cancer, please be patient, tolerant and loving. If they are experiencing some of the horrific financial difficulties that seem to accompany this disease, help in any way you can. I have tried not to complain about my disease to others but sometimes that just becomes a daunting task. I will say that no one knows what I have really been through, not even my children. For the better part of this they were too young to even understand. Most of the time I felt I was all alone in my battle. Emotional support was all but absent most of the time. It seems no-one wants to be around sick people. Maybe it makes them realize just how vulnerable we are to illness and disease. For those of you out there with this disease, read on and SURVIVE! Take my hand and let us walk together.

CHAPTER I

My First Encounter with Death

I debated whether or not to include the first two chapters in this book because they really have nothing to do with Cancer. I include them only as a testimony to two things. First they help to show the development of my spiritual self and how that affected my prognosis. These incidences helped open the door for how my own spiritual being began to grow dramatically. It also attests to the resilience of the human body and the strength of the human spirit in the face of insurmountable odds. GOD MADE US STRONG! I am going to keep the first part of this book focused on my medical history in an attempt to show what a person can endure if the desire to survive is there and strong enough. I will expand on my own feelings concerning Spirituality, Philosophy and Theology later in the book and as the title says, a few other thoughts to ponder.

My first real experience with illness came when I got married for the second time. Of course I had experienced the usual colds and flu when I was growing up. I had few problems with strep throat but certainly nothing that would ever be considered life threatening. About a week before our wedding, I began to experience some pain in my chest. I went to my doctor who had been a friend of mine for several years. We were both former Marines and even attended the annual Marine Corps Birthday bash together a few times. He listened to my chest for quite a while. He told me he thought I had a touch of Pleurisy. Pleurisy is an inflammation of the tissue surrounding the lungs. He said the inflammation was what was causing the pain in my chest. He prescribed an anti-inflammatory medication. I took the prescription and within a few days, the pain subsided. I was getting married that Sunday and we were having the rehearsal dinner that Saturday night. I did not sleep well Friday night and woke up about four in the morning in terrible pain. I was coughing very hard and very deep. Every time I coughed it felt like someone was plunging a hot knife into my lungs. I got out of bed and called my doctor's service. A few minutes later a doctor called me and told me my doctor was on vacation and he was filling in for him. He then asked me how he could help me. I informed him of my condition and he told me if the pain was that severe I needed to get to the hospital. He said he would meet us there. Now remember, I have a rehearsal dinner that evening.

When we got to the ER the doctor was already there. They took my temperature and it was 104. He listened to my chest and I am pretty sure at this point he had his own suspicions about what it was, but I believe he was holding off until he knew for sure. He told me they were going to do some X-Rays to see if that would indicate the problem. After the X-Rays I lay in the ER waiting. I was in terrible pain. I just could not seem to quit coughing and every time I coughed it hurt tremendously. He soon returned and he had a nurse and a hospital administrator with him. He then proceeded to tell me I had the worst case of pneumonia he had ever seen in his twenty three years of practicing medicine. He told me they needed to get me admitted immediately. "Whoa!" I said. I told him I was getting married the next day and had a rehearsal dinner that evening. By the look on his face I think he thought I possibly did not understand the seriousness of my condition. I told him to just give me a big shot of penicillin in the butt and some pain medication and I would report back right after the wedding the next day. He did not like that at all. He was trying desperately to get me admitted but I was not listening. My total focus was on the wedding and the dinner. He tried to employ my wife as an advocate for his point of view. Finally after much discussion I told him I was leaving one way or another. As he was giving me the shot he was behind me mumbling about how what he was doing was paramount to malpractice. I told him not to worry I was not going to sue him and chuckled. I do not think he found it very funny though. I just wanted to get the wedding over with then I would deal with this.

My soon to be wife and I left the hospital and she was not too happy with what I had done. She told me she knew I was a big tough Marine and all that but this could kill me! I was sweating like a stuck pig all day. They had given me some medication at hospital to help but I was still in a tremendous amount of pain. The day seemed to go on forever. I tried to get some sleep and rest my body for the events that evening but could not sleep. I tossed and turned and was soak and wet. Finally my wife to be told me it was time to get ready for the dinner. My whole body was sweating profusely. I took my temperature and it was still 104. I threw down 800mg of Ibuprofen and a pain med. That evening we went to the dinner but said nothing to anyone about my illness. I just kept joking about being nervous when anyone made a comment about me sweating so much. I managed to get through the dinner but my best man and I had been friends since we were kids and he knew something was not quite right. I had to tell him. He was astonished and got very angry with me and went on a rant about how stubborn I was and all that. I told him his ranting would do no good, I was determined to make the wedding happen the next day.

The next day we had our wedding at the beautiful Botanical Gardens downtown. Getting ready for the wedding ceremony was an enormous task. I was still sweating and clothes clung to me. Imagine putting on a Tuxedo in the shower and you can get the picture of how I felt. When we got there, my wife to be looked stunning and I almost forgot I was sick for a while. The wedding ceremony went perfectly other than the fact that I was soaked and looked like death warmed over. I remember the vows seemed to take forever. The pastor pronounced us man and wife and we kissed. It was a very long kiss. Everyone clapped and we turned and smiled.

At this point my wife and I as well as the wedding party lined up for the usual hand shaking and congratulations. As the guests exited the area we were in, they would turn to the left and walk down a hall to the vehicles waiting outside. Just outside, the limousine and other wedding procession vehicles were parked. Everyone was waiting for the bride and groom to exit for the usual throwing the rice and so on. There was only one problem, no bride and groom were coming out. What happened next caught them all by surprise. No one except my best man knew I was sick. As the last couple passed to leave the wedding area I remember following them with my eyes as they rounded the corner. As they walked down the hall my eyes rolled up into the back of my head and I went straight over backwards. I was unconscious. Everyone was in a panic. My best man scooped me up and they loaded me into the back of the limousine. People were confused and astonished. Many had already left for the reception and would not find out what had happened until later. I regained consciousness for a brief time and told my wife to go and get the reception started. The limo driver was thoroughly confused by all this and when my best man told him to head for the hospital it caught him completely by surprise and I was told later he had responded to the order, "The Hospital"? My best man looked at me and said, "A groom-less wedding reception, only you Ace, only you. Ace was his nickname for me.

We arrived at the hospital and I was unconscious again. Now try and picture this. A white stretch limo pulls up to the Emergency Room entrance and you see them pull a guy in a white tuxedo out, load him on a gurney, and run him inside. Most curious I would say. Those who did see probably thought the groom had a bit too much to drink or something like that. The next thing I remember was being in a hospital bed with all kinds of tubes running out of me. Breathing was extremely difficult and my upper body was in great pain. A doctor came in and told me I had the most advanced case of pneumonia he had ever seen (different doctor). They were pushing antibiotics, saline and God knows what into my system in an effort to keep me alive. At some point people started coming up from the reception to visit me. They would not let the really drunk ones in.

Everyone was astonished at the events of the evening. Lots of stories were told about the reception and I remember several men offering to consummate my marriage for me. There was even this rumor down at the nurses' station that a man was dying and it was his last wish to marry this woman on his deathbed. How romantic I thought. But there was no romance that night. I also remember my dad standing next to the bed holding my hand....crying. It was the only time I had ever seen my father cry but I was pretty sure I knew why. He had a brother named Bill who died in his early twenties from pneumonia. This was obviously bringing back some bad memories. I was in and out a lot that night. I do remember there was a great deal of activity in the room though.

At some point I must have passed out. Or so you would have thought. The next thing I knew, there was a guy with a set of defibrillator paddles in his hands standing over me. I looked up at him and said, "This can't be good". He seemed astonished that I could talk and was coherent. He said, "I had to pop you twice to get you back, you were flat-lined for forty two seconds". Oh my God, I was dead for forty two seconds I thought. Many people who know this part of the story have asked me if I saw the bright lights or God or any of that. But I had not. I did know God was there looking after me though, or I would not be alive. I told them not to call my wife as I was alright and I knew she had to work the next day. I also made the doctor promise not to tell her what had happened as she was already worried enough. Every day was long and intense. There were medications, breathing exercises and the constant checking of vital signs looking for any change in my condition. Even though I was not a very spiritual person at this point in my life, I still prayed. I was fighting with everything I had in me. I soon discovered that even though you are very ill, there is no sleeping for any length of time in a hospital. People were coming and going constantly, all having some vital role in your continued existence. I think they give you the drugs just to keep your sanity through these kinds of ordeals.

Several days passed but I did not seem to be getting any better. My wife worked during the day and then would come up at night and stay until she was too tired to take it anymore. She was scared and worried. On the fourth or fifth morning my regular doctor came in. I asked him if he had enjoyed his vacation. He immediately started into a lecture about how he could not believe that I had refused to be admitted and how I had put my life at risk. I was too weak to argue with him. A short time later another doctor came into the room. He was a surgeon. They both proceeded to tell me that my condition had worsened and I was now past the pneumonia stage and now had a disease known as Empyema. Empyema is when the fluid from the pneumonia perforates the walls of the lungs and starts seeping through and collecting on the outside of the lug. He said he was pretty sure I was the first case of Empyema in that hospital since the thirties. He said people just did not get that sick anymore with the antibiotics of modern day medicine, and if they did, they usually died. That was a nice thought. I know I certainly felt like I was dying! They were listening to my heart and seemed amazed at how strong the beat was. They told me they wanted to perform a procedure known as a Thorensentesis. This involved taking a syringe that looked like it was meant to be used on a horse and inserting into my chest cavity and drawing the fluid out that had collected outside the lung. They scheduled the procedure for the next morning as they wanted me to rest a little more before they did it.

The next morning the surgeon and two nurses came in with a cart loaded down with a syringe and surgical instruments. They had me sit on the edge of the bed and the second nurse stood in front of me so I could rest my hands on her shoulders to keep my arms elevated. The doctor told me he was going to give me a local anesthetic. He told me he would then make a small incision to slide the needle through. My God, the needle was so big they had to slit you first to put it in! I could feel a pushing sensation as he slid the needle into my back. He made the comment that I had the thickest rib bones he had ever seen. He seemed surprised as I am not a very big man. Suddenly I felt very intense pain. The nurse whose shoulders my hands were resting on suddenly went to the floor as my grip on her quickly tightened and I pushed her to the floor and she was crying. I was apologizing over and over for hurting her. She told me that was not the reason she was crying. I looked confused and she said she would tell me later. The pain was still excruciating. The other nurse and the doctor were still behind me but I could not see them. They were whispering and I could hear and feel a lot of movement behind me. They finally finished. The pain was still horrible and asked the doctor what happened. He said he would explain it to me later after the procedure.

In came another nurse with a small syringe in her hand. She injected it into my IV tube and I soon felt the pain subsiding very quickly. Mmmmmm, I was thinking. I asked her what she had given me and she said a shot of Demerol. Long live Demerol I was thinking. A little while later the other nurse who had been crying returned and told me what had happened. She proceeded to tell me that when the doctor had inserted the needle my lateral muscles had contracted and the needle had either broken or bent and the pain I felt was it scoring the wall of my lung. She said she knew it must have been terribly painful and that was why she had the tears in her eyes. The surgeon repeated the same procedure three more times, minus the bent needle of course. He went in twice through my back and once under my arm. I remember fighting for my life every day. "I am too young to die" I was thinking. They did tests and took X-Rays several times a day.

The next couple of days were rather uneventful but it was apparent that things were very intense. Meanwhile my wife worried and cried. It was the waiting game as they ran bag after bag of antibiotics through me. Everyone was trying to cheer me up. Friends were telling all those jokes about me being too ornery to die and all that. Finally one morning as I awoke, I realized I felt a little better. The next day a little better yet. That morning my doctor came in and sat on the edge of the bed and told me my fever was dropping and he thought I was on my way to recovery. As he sat on the edge of the bed, he held my hand and said, "I could not tell you before because I did not want you to give up, but I thought you were going to die every day for the first week". He told me it was my strong heart that had saved me. He told my wife it looked like I was going to be alright and I am not sure I had ever seen her smile so big. He also said if I ever pulled stupid stunt like this again, referring to not letting myself be admitted in the first place that HE would kill me! Finally after five more days, the doctor came in and told me they were going to release me. I took a little time off and then it was back to work. At this time in my life I was still not able to appreciate what had just happened to me. How quickly we move on when we are young. I did not know it but God had just given me what would turn out to be the second of many chances to live again.

CHAPTER II

My Second Encounter with Death

A few years later my wife and I met a man that would change my life forever. In some ways this would prove to be good and in some ways bad. He claimed he was a Christian but his life was obsessed with politics and he was very bitter. It was not that anything he was telling me had anything to do with spirituality, but it led me there eventually. It was at that time that I really began to look at my own spirituality. I was reading the Bible a little and searching for some answers to some things. I was also starting to pray more and was spending a great deal of time contemplating philosophy and what our life is all about. I have grown so much since then. God uses different ways and things to teach each of us. This man had opened the door to my own search and I am sure he had no idea he had done it. The information he had given me created an overwhelming sense of curiosity and thirst for knowledge that are to this day the single greatest motivator to expanding my spirituality. The only thing that was important was that I was searching.

Now for the second story. When I was younger, I had a bit of a drinking problem. I did not drink often but when I did, look out. One Friday night my wife was going out with the girls so I decided to go out too. I do not know if you have ever heard the song by George Thorogood called "I drink Alone" but that was the perfect description of how I did it. I drank way to much that night. In fact I did not have any idea how drunk I was. I then climbed into my car and proceeded to head for home. As I was driving down the street I approached the intersection of Broadway and Main. They had recently re-paved Broadway and tried to feather the fresh asphalt out onto Main. This left an enormous dip on the two corners where the storm drains were located on both sides. I hit the first dip and almost lost control of my car. Then I hit the second dip but was still recovering from the surprise of the first. I lost control of the wheel and the right front tire jumped up onto the curb. About a foot from the edge of the curb was a support cable that went up to a nearby telephone pole. The wishbone on the wheel of my car got caught on the cable and up it went. To this day I cannot figure out how things happened as they did. I was only going thirty-five miles per hour or so.

The car was caught on the cable and propelled right up it. I remember to this day going wheeeeeeee as I was rising up in the air like a little kid on a roller coaster. Drunk does as drunk is you know. The next thing that happened was the car rolled over twice in the air and came down upside down in the middle of the street with me facing traffic. I did not know it at the time, but somewhere behind was a gentleman in a Chevrolet Blazer. He could not stop and he T-Boned my vehicle as I lay upside down in the street and I was sucking the chrome off his bumper. The impact knocked me unconscious. I regained consciousness and was lying on the top of the inside of the vehicle. At that time, I did not even know there was another vehicle involved. The car was upside down. The top of the car was crushed down to the top of the seats and head rests were bent over and I was trapped inside. The steering column was pushed about eight inches into the dashboard and there was glass everywhere. The main support post on my side of the car was pushed in almost to the middle of the car. I was in a great deal of pain and that pain was all over my body. I was pretty sure I had broken my neck and a couple of ribs at the very least. I did not move as I knew that may just add to my injuries. It seemed so quiet and serene considering the circumstances. But I guess at three-thirty in the morning, it usually is.

What happened next caught me totally off guard. This is where things started to get a little weird. A woman's voice suddenly said,

"How bad are you hurt?" Now I knew I had been alone in the car. There is no way this woman could have gotten into the car from what I was seeing but there she was right over the top of me. I asked her who she was. Fortunately for me, the accident happened about a thousand feet from the Emergency Room entrance to the Catholic Hospital downtown. She told me she was a nurse who had just got off work and was standing just inside the ER entrance when the crash occurred talking to a friend. She told me there was an ambulance on the way. I told her I thought my neck was broken and a couple of ribs too. She asked me if I could move my fingers and toes. I wiggled my toes and fingers and told her yes. She said she doubted that my neck was broken. Then, she disappeared as quickly as she had appeared. I know I did not imagine this woman and I have never hallucinated on alcohol. I thought she must have crawled out the same way she came in and I just could not see where that was. A short time later I could hear the sirens. I heard truck doors slamming and voices. The next thing I knew there was a fireman outside asking if anyone was alive. I answered yes and then they started up the chop saws.

It took two crews of firemen forty-five minute to cut me out of the car with chop saws and the infamous "Jaws of Life". Finally the door came off and there they were! I told them I thought my neck was broken so they brought out a board to put me on. I asked where the nurse was that had been inside my car. They thought I was referring to a passenger. I said no that a woman had climbed inside the car while I was waiting for them arrive and had just crawled back out right before they got there. The fireman said he doubted that. He told me the top of the car was crushed down so far that there was no way anyone could have gotten in or out. They said no one was there but me and the guy in the Blazer behind me that had T-Boned my car and he was also unconscious. He said that they had seen no one as they approached the accident either. That's weird I thought because I knew she was a nurse and would never have left me there knowing I was so badly hurt. They put me in the ambulance and drove me to the Emergency Room entrance about a thousand feet away. Shortest Ambulance ride in history probably.

As I was wheeled inside they put me face down on yet another board that had a hole cut out for my face and another board on my back and strapped me down to immobilize me. They would rotate me like a chicken on a spit every so often. I was told that was so all the blood did not rush to one side. They were also working on getting my lung re-inflated. I was not breathing very well. As soon as they got me stabilized they ran me up to X-ray. They took lots and lots of X-Rays. When I was done, I was taken back to the Emergency Room ICU. By this time, my wife was there and was frantic. As she had been coming down Main Street to the hospital she had seen my car crushed and upside down on a flatbed truck going the other way. She was horrified by what she saw on that truck. We had just had our first child six months earlier. The most beautiful little girl you ever saw. What I saw next scared the hell out of me. She was standing next to a priest. The priest walked over to me and I totally lost it. I remembered my time in the service and the only time the priest came was if you were going to die! I became frantic and uncontrollable at that point. He walked back over to my wife and said, "I don't think he was very happy to see me". I screamed at my wife to divorce me because they would take all our money for the medical bills. I was a raving lunatic at that point I guess. Apparently someone else thought I was being a little crazy too because a man came over and gave me shot which seemed to calm me down considerably.

A little later a doctor walked up to me with a feather in his hand. Now this was strange, a doctor walking around with a feather in his hand. He leaned over and ran the feather along the bottoms of my feet, my legs, arms, fingers and a number of other places. He kept asking me if I could feel that and I kept telling him yes. He looked very confused and ordered the nurse to take me back to X-Ray. After what seemed an eternity, two doctors approached me. One was a neurologist. They told me I had broken the first two Cervical Vertebrae in my neck. I had broken what is called the "Dens of the Axis" clean off and it was wedged between the front of the vertebrae and the spinal cord. They seemed to be very confused how I still had feeling in my arms, legs or at all for that matter. They said that from what they were seeing on the X-Rays, I should be a quadriplegic. No feeling anywhere except the head. They told me my spinal cord had been severely traumatized by the impact. They also told me I had four broken ribs, two in front and two in back. In addition to that, I had crushed my left lung, my spleen and one of my kidneys. The latter two were seeping fluid and they seemed very concerned.

Years later, I found out I had also broken my hip. Guess there was so much concern for other life threatening issues they must have missed that one. What a mess I was I thought. I began to pray wondering if I was going to make it through the night or ever walk again. I had been extremely athletic most of my life and the thought of suddenly being a quadriplegic just terrified me. I am sure the alcohol was not helping the anxiety either. The broken ribs and crushed lungs were from having pushed the steering column eight inches into the dash board with my chest. I imagine the broken neck was from the top of the car crushing down onto me. I guess I will never know. Again I have to ask, "More luck or coincidence?" Another save for the Lord I think.

As I lay there between the boards I had a lot of waiting to do so I inquired about the nurse who had crawled into the car with me. I thought for sure since I was right where this woman said she worked, someone would know who she was. I wanted to thank her. I thought she was incredibly brave and very much a credit to the nursing profession. In addition to all the broken glass which she could easily have cut herself on, there was gas everywhere and that car could have caught fire and blew up and any moment. Yet again no one seemed to know who I was talking about. No nurses or even the shift supervisor. Later I even contacted the hospital director and made an inquiry. He told me he would do some checking and get back to me. A few days later he called me and said that he could not find anyone who knew who this woman could possibly have been. He was pretty sure she was not one of his nurses.

At this point I think it would be appropriate to tell you something my mother shared with me years ago. My mother was a very spiritual person most of her life. Years ago my mother contracted Colorectal

Cancer and needed to have surgery. She was put in the hospital the night before awaiting the surgery early the next morning. She told me she was scared and experiencing a great deal of anxiety over the upcoming surgery. She told me she had been unable to sleep and was awake in her bed. She then said that as she lay there, a light suddenly appeared next to her bed. Then an angel materialized and told her not to worry, that everything was going to be alright. She said that she then KNEW she was going to be alright and felt a great wave of calm come over herself. I guess divine intervention runs in the family. Even though I think such events of spirituality are extremely rare, I have never doubted my mother's story. I later found out she had never told this story to anyone in the family other than me. Not even my father or my one sister whom she told everything. Hmmmmmmm again. I never thought about it until later, but I cannot help but wonder if my Nurse was an angel too.

There is another aspect of this story that has always puzzled me too. It was winter and I was wearing a very thick suede jacket with a sheepskin lining that night. The sleeve of that jacket had been cut clean from the shoulder hem all the way to the cuff and was hanging loose at my side. The cut was so clean it looked as if it had been made with a razor. Not a frayed edge anywhere. I guess at the time I just figured it was cut by glass somehow during the accident. It did not occur to me until later that there was not a single scratch or cut on my arm anywhere. Is this more luck or coincidence? As you can see, at some point here you have to ask yourself just how much luck or coincidence or whatever you would like to call it had occurred in my life. And as you will see there is much more to come. What is it they say about God taking care of fools?

Eventually they got me stabilized and moved me to a room. Again I found myself in a hospital bed with a lot of tubes running out of me. They had managed to re-inflate my left lung and I was breathing much better. There was still a fair amount of seepage around the spleen and kidney though and they seemed concerned. They also came in to wrap my ribs which I guess is about all they can do. One of the following days my doctor and a neurosurgeon came to visit. The surgeon explained in more detail what had happened to the vertebrae in my neck and seemed to be very confused by the lack of any paralysis. They were taking X-Rays almost daily to monitor any changes. A few days later, the surgeon told me the swelling in my neck had gone down considerably and that the dens of the axis bone had come free. He told me he wanted to try and reset the bone using a medical device called a Halo. I told him I knew what it was because I had seen a show on television that talked about it. A Halo is a device that is used to immobilize the head and keep it straight.

The device consists of a shoulder mount, four upright rods and a band of metal covered by cloth that fits around your head almost like a sweatband you would wear for exercising. In the headband are four places where hardened thumb screws thread through. These screws are ground to a point and are actually screwed right into the skull. They administer a local anesthetic, make all the proper adjustments and then they tighten the screws. What I heard next was one of the most mind shaking things I have ever heard in my life. Even though you really did not feel the screws as they turned them in, you did HEAR them as they went into your skull. It is a sound I will never forget. They then make some final adjustments. If all this was not bad enough, I was going to have to wear this thing for the next three months. It also meant I was going to have to sleep on my back which was not how I normally slept. This made sleeping very difficult for the next three months.

I was finally released from the hospital a few weeks later. It seemed I had dodged some very high caliber bullets here. There is no place like home I thought as I walked through the front door of my house. We had bought a used hospital bed and put it in the family room next to the sliding patio doors. It was February and it was snowing a lot. The view was beautiful. I love the fresh snow. It covers up all the filth and makes the world look so clean for a while. Snow is just more of the beauty of God's creation. The doctor had given me a prescription for Hydrocodone for the pain. That is not what they used at the hospital but as long as it dealt with the pain I did not really care. A short time after taking the first dose of it, I was starting to hear, see and feel very strange things. The next thing I knew, I was in a total panic attack seeing myself trapped inside the car again. I then jumped up, threw open the patio doors and ran out into the snow. I was standing in the middle of my back yard in snow up to my knees in a pair of shorts panting like a dog on a hot summer's day. It was a horrible feeling as I was reliving the accident except this time I was not drunk! We called the doctor and he said that it was probably an allergic reaction to the Hydrocodone. My wife had a few Percosets left from her Cicerian Section and they seemed to work much better.

A halo is a very strange thing to get used to. Almost everything in your life suddenly becomes much different. As I was taking a shower one day, I leaned over to wash my legs and put one of the halo rods right through the fiberglass molded shower in our bathroom. At the next appointment we were discussing some of these types of things and one of the nurses said that many people take balls and mount them to the ends of the rods. So we went to store and found some very colorful Nerf Balls and mounted them to the end of the rods. They were also fluorescent and you could see me coming a mile away. Sleeping was probably the most difficult part of it for me. The bulkiness of the halo made it extremely hard to get comfortable and the pain was not helping either.

My daughter was only about seven months old at this time. She would try to hug me or kiss me as she would sit on the bed with me and kept bumping her head on the halo. It would hurt and she would cry. She soon decided not to kiss daddy anymore. It broke my heart. My wife worked during the day and I would take care of the baby. My wife was very unhappy about the fact that I was so drunk and how all this had happened because of it. I was not working and it would also be quite some time before I could which of course put the entire burden of our finances onto her. A short time later, my wife's mother died. She left my wife some money and that in combination with my wife's earnings is what kept the boat afloat. By the time it was all over, she had spent all of her inheritance paying bills and was not happy about that either. The evening of the accident, the local news was there and she had managed to get a copy of the film from one of the local channels. She has also gone to the junk yard and taken pictures of the car. I had not seen it since the accident. What I saw left me breathless. I looked at the crushed hunk of metal all twisted and crushed in several places and came to realize that God must truly love me. There is no way someone should have ever left that vehicle alive. My faith started to grow. I still have those pictures and open them on occasion to remind myself of just how much he does.

A few months passed and it was time to find out if the halo had worked. I met the doctor and they did some X-Rays to see if the bone had rest itself. This was very interesting to see. X-Rays in real time is amazing to me. There was nothing but disappointment for me that day though. As I tilted my head slightly forward I watched the bone jump a little. I looked at the doctor and he said we should head back to his office to discuss my options. I was thinking to myself at least I had options! My wife was very quiet as we drove. The doctor then began to explain my options. The first one was to do nothing and someday I may turn my head or be impacted and suddenly find myself paralyzed. Not really an option I thought. The second was to have a procedure known as a C-1/C-2 Fusion. It would be a very high risk surgery he told us. He explained that they would make an incision from the middle of the back of my head down to the upper part of my back. Then they would retract the neck muscles and remove the bone. I still have never been able to figure out how they accomplished that without taking the vertebrae apart. Then they go into your lower back and break off a piece of bone and grind it down to fit between the vertebrae. They place it between the first two vertebrae and clamp the three bones together using screws and straps. After a period of time, the bones would encapsulate with new bone and they basically become one thus creating the "fusion" of the C-1 and the C-2 vertibrae. There would some loss of movement but it would probably be minimal. I would also still be living in bed for another four months. As we were walking down the hall I asked the doctor when he wanted to do it and he told me to talk to the scheduling nurse. My wife was flabbergasted. She asked me, "How can you make decision like that so quickly?" I told her I really did not see any other option. My wife also seemed very concerned about how young she thought the surgeon looked and wondered if he was qualified to even do this. I must say he did have a bit of a baby face. His name was Dr. Dozier and my wife called him Doogie Dozier in reference to the television show.

By this time in my life, I was thinking a lot more about my spirituality. Events had got me to thinking. There were some other totally unrelated events that had occurred during this period of my life that were also pointing me in that direction. I began to pray and wanted to spend some time reading the bible which was kind of hard to do considering at this point I did not even own one. I was beginning to understand a little something about faith in God. He obviously loved me and cared for me, otherwise I would not be here. I remember being very scared when we reported for the surgery. I was gripping my wife's hand tightly and praying in my mind. This would be the first real surgery I had ever had other than having my tonsils out. I was scared that morning. They were preparing me for surgery and gave me a shot of morphine which helped to calm me. The surgery lasted eleven hours. I woke up in a hospital bed and immediately sat up and started high projectile vomiting. I had fluid running down the back of my neck which I was sure was blood. I managed to reach down and grab a trash can and started to fill it. A nurse came in and was not very happy I was vomiting into her trash can. She handed me a little silver pan and said to do it in there. At that moment I leaned over blasting another round into the trash can. She got very angry and I looked at her and said, "Do you REALLY think that will hold what I am doing here?" She walked out of the room and said to do it in the pan. I mumbled a few choice words at her and filled the can some more. The doctor later told me I was so sick because of the length of the surgery and the anesthesia.

Later as I lay there, I felt the back of my head. It was shaved and I could feel an incision about 8 or 9 inches long running vertically down the middle of my head and back. There were two other lateral incisions that were about an inch log where I imagine drain tubes had been. I was told that the surgery had gone well and the doctor was very optimistic about my recovery. He said I was young and very strong. I always try to be optimistic about things so if there was a silver lining to all this, my being home meant I would get to spend a great deal of the next four months with my baby girl. I would sing to her and hold her in my arms. We would dance and laugh. They were such wonderful memories at a time of such pain. She was probably the best therapy I could have ever received at the time. I would end up spending about 7 or 8 months of my life in that hospital bed. Eight months of my life lost because I just did not know when to go home. It was one of life's EXTREME lessons.

I have not even drank a beer now for almost twenty years. I guess at least I learned that lesson. They did come and arrest me for DUI nine months later though. The day the warrant was to expire. There was nothing a judge could do that could compare to what I had been through. I was convicted of DUI anyways. Lying in that bed all that time had given me a lot of time to think and reflect though. Little did I know what was to come some years later. I saw myself getting better and better and my mind drifted from some of the lessons I had learned. They were quickly forgotten. Out of sight, out of mind as the saying goes. No Wisdom yet.

It was not long after that I was able to go back to work. Things were going well and we were quickly outgrowing our house with the new baby. We found a beautiful house that had even been a Parade of Homes house when it was built. It seemed like a castle in comparison to where we were living. We had quite a bit of equity in our current home and were able to make a very large down payment. This made getting a loan for the new house much easier. We got a fantastic deal on it and were very excited. We had to buy quite a bit of new furniture as it was so much larger than the old house. Almost three times the size. It suddenly seemed that maybe some of life's problems had passed. Then suddenly one day I went to work only to find the company I worked for was letting people go. I lost my job. Here we had just bought this house and all this furniture and I was unemployed. I could feel the panic mode returning. I managed to find a job as a manger of a local tobacco shop close to my house. It did not pay much but it kept the bills paid if I worked enough. I was a smoker and knew a great many of my customers. It seems fate is not without a strange sense of irony. I was managing a tobacco shop and then I would later get Cancer. I was also spreading the ill effects of smoking to all my customers. That job did not last long though.

As a teenager I had worked for several builders and when I got out of the service I had owned a small contracting business as I was going to college. When we moved in I was constantly doing some type of improvements to the house. I was constantly installing something new such as new windows, doors, a fence and so on. As I was putting up the fence one day, one of my neighbors stopped. I guess he assumed I was a contractor and asked me if I would give him an estimate on something he wanted done. I then told him I was not a contractor I was his new neighbor. He was embarrassed. I guess I have that contractor look. Later that evening I was telling my wife about what had happened. I thought it was amusing. As I told her I could see the look in her eyes and knew the gears were turning. She then asked me, "Why don't you go back into contracting again? I was apprehensive and asked her if she knew how long it would take to get a business going to the point of being able to pay the bills. She asked me what I had to loose. She did have a point.

The next day we printed up some little three fold flyers and I went around to all of my neighbors' homes and slipped one in their doors. I have always loved working with my hands and had the skills to do this. A few days later the phone rang and I got my first job. To make long story short, I did not leave my neighborhood for the next seven months. I was also developing several relationships with the new home improvement store that had just opened. There were a lot of builders that did business there. Word was quickly getting around about the quality of my work and before I knew it, some of these builders were also calling me. My business took off so fast I could not keep up. We were doing very well at this point and even bought onto a time share. We were living large as they say these days. Little did I know what was about to happen a few years later.

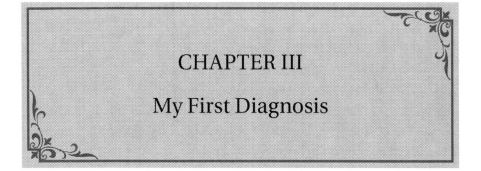

CHAPTER III

My First Diagnosis

I did not join the Veteran's Administration Health Care System until I had been out of the service for many years. I had always thought that you had to either be retired from the service or have a service related injury to get care through the VA. One day I saw a friend of mine and as we were talking he said something about going to the VA to pick up some medication. I knew he had been in the Navy but was only in two years and was never injured during his service. I then asked him how he was doing this. He told me that in 1996 the Congress had opened the VA Health Care System to anyone who had two years of continuous active service and an Honorable Discharge. I have a seizure disorder and my medication was costing me almost one hundred dollars a month and I did not have any health insurance. He told me the medication would only cost me seven dollars a month there. The next day I went to the local VA hospital and was told I would have to apply first. I filled out all the necessary forms and waited for the reply. A short time later I was thrilled to find I had been accepted into the program but needed to set up and appointment to be assigned a Primary Care Physician. A short time later I received a little card in the mail telling me when my first appointment was. I was thrilled just to be saving the ninety-three dollars a month on my medication. Little did I know that I would soon be facing a rather extensive evaluation so they could assess my health care needs.

I was a type B Hepatitis carrier and had been taking medication for my seizure disorder for many years and they were a little concerned about the effects that may have had on my liver. I went for several tests and things seemed to be moving right along. In 2004 I went for an appointment with my doctor. He had noticed there was no family medical history in the computer and then asked me several questions about my family medical history so he could put it into the computer. When I mentioned my mother had been diagnosed with Colorectal Cancer several years ago and had a Colostomy he stopped and asked me how old I was. He then asked me if I had ever had a Colonoscopy. I told him no that it had not exactly been on the top of my list of things to do. He stressed the importance of me getting one as Colon Cancer can be hereditary. They did a gene test to see if I had the BRCA gene mutation.

He stressed the importance of scheduling the test. He also told me that half the men that schedule one, never show up. Some kind of crazy mental thing about being gay or something I imagine. I told him I would schedule the test and I would show up. I really did not give it much thought as I was in extremely good shape for my age. I was a contractor and my job was very physical as you can imagine. People used to ask me if I worked out and would say, "Work out? Who needs to work out, I got a job!" I made the appointment for the Colonoscopy and received my prep. The prep was two bottles of liquid you drank at certain intervals which causes bowel movements and empties out the entire gastro-intestinal system. I had not even thought about that the fact that the colon would have to be emptied so they can see in there. So I went home and took the prep, and empty I did. Alllll night long! Even a drink of water sent me running for the bathroom. Eventually my system calmed down and I was able to sleep.

I reported for my procedure the next morning. The doctor explained to me what they would be doing to me that day. First they administer the anesthetic. It was called "Conscious Sedation". They knock you out but not all the way. You do not really know what is going on but you are able to respond to them. The only thing I remember was that the doctor kept saying, "You are moving again Mr. Flick". Then they started the actual procedure. They pump air through your rectum into your colon to enlarge it. Then they take a scope and a light that is mounted on a long flexible tube and slide it inside you and look for abnormalities in the colon. It also had a camera on it so they can take pictures of anything they find. Later when I viewed the pictures I was amazed at what it looked like in there. It was not at all like I had pictured in my mind. A very ingenious device I thought. It never ceases to amaze me what man has invented to get the job done.

Prior to the procedure I was told that when I woke up I would be in a room used for recovery and my wife and kids would be there. They also said they would discuss the results of the test at that time. When I came to, I looked around and all seemed well. I was awake, felt fine, and was in what seemed to be an area that would be used for recovery. Everything seemed copasetic. I said, "Hello, I'm awake". The curtain swung aside and a nurse came in. I looked around and realized I was not where I was supposed to be. I was in the Intensive Care Unit (ICU). The nurse told me there had been a problem with my heart during the test. From what I could understand, your heartbeat has a primary and secondary point of origin from where your heartbeat originates. For some reason mine had jumped over to the secondary during the test. It had now returned to the primary but they just wanted to make sure everything was alright. About that time, my wife and kids came in. I am always happy to see my children. Their smiles make the pressures of life wisp away to be replaced by great joy. The nurse came in and told me I could get dressed and leave. Since no one had said anything was wrong, I figured I had passed the test with flying colors. I was still a little groggy from the sedation and I guess I did not take note of the look on my wife's face.

My wife had to drive as I was still under the effects of the sedation. I remember leaving the hospital and as we were driving away saying to my wife, "Well everything must have been ok or they would have said something". She turned her head quickly and looked at me, her mouth wide open. She then looked back at the road. She looked surprised and shocked at the same time. She did this several times before the words blurted out. "They didn't tell you?" There was a look of fear and despair in her eyes. "You have Cancer!" she said. She said the doctor told her I had a growth right above the rectum. It was very low he had said. She said that he had told her he knew Cancer when he saw it. I do not know if I was in denial or the fact that my wife had a knack for being a little emotional in her responses to things, but I remember being very calm. I told her I was sure they would have to run a biopsy to determine that and not to get all worked up about it yet. I cannot be sure because we were not the best communicators but I am sure there were some thoughts of her childhood at that point. Her father was a smoker and had died of Lung Cancer when she was sixteen.... and I smoked. I think to this day she thinks all my Cancer was caused by my smoking.

We had nearly separated several times due to my smoking. I am not really sure if the kids had known at that point, but if they did not, they did now because mom just blurted it out in front of them. I found out later that it had scared the hell out of them. I tried to reassure them that they would need to do some more tests to find out what he had seen. They told me later the only thing they had heard was mom say dad had Cancer. They spent a lot of time in their rooms that night crying and worrying they told me they told me years later. I remember my son asking me if I was going to die. I told him God would take care of me and not to worry. My children were quite young at that time. My daughter was six and my son was three. Both were extremely smart for their ages and knew something was up even if daddy was trying to act like nothing serious was wrong.

I soon received a call from the VA to schedule an appointment to have the biopsy done. Again, my wife had to drive for the same reasons. The difference was, this time the appointment was in Indianapolis at the Roudebush Medical Center, the main VA hospital in Indiana. We had to stay overnight as the procedure was early the next morning. I was pleasantly surprised to find out that the VA provided lodging very nearby. We did not talk a lot that night as I think we were both a little preoccupied with what the next day may bring. I was also spending a lot of time in the bathroom as I had to go through the same preparation routine as before. We got there and again they explained the test and the sedation. It was a little different this time though. When he inserted the device this time, I was very much conscious. I was amazed as I could watch everything he was doing on a television monitor to my left. I was not feeling anything, but I could see it. He slid in the tubing that the camera and light were mounted on, but this one also had some kind of little tool on the end. He knew exactly where to go because of the previous test and went immediately to the spot. There it was! Right before my very eyes! The growth the doctor had found during the Colonoscopy. The device he was controlling had a set of what looked like tiny clam shells on the end facing each other that came together. He made a pass and removed about a third of the tumor. He would then repeat the same thing two more times and the tumor appeared to be gone except for what looked like a little scar on the colon wall. Each time, he would pull the device out and place the tissue in a Petrie dish to be biopsied later.

As we were on our way home that afternoon, I think it was finally starting to occur to me that something may actually be wrong. I think I stayed relatively calm but there was obviously some anxiety involved. Then we had to wait for what seemed to be an eternity for the results. I also went online and did some reading on the subject. I was not totally unfamiliar with Colorectal Cancer because as I said, my mother had it. She had a procedure known as a Colostomy. A Colostomy is a procedure that saves a great many people from dying of Colon Cancer. First, they remove the Cancerous portion of the colon. That length of colon that is removed depends on any number of variables. Then they suture or glue your rear end shut. Wow, there goes the toilet paper bill! Last, but not least, they make an incision in your lower left abdomen. They then bring about a one inch length of the end of the colon, called a stoma, out through your abdomen and attached it. It forms a seal and from that point forward, that is where your stool exits the body. No more number two so to say.

Now obviously you cannot just have a bowel movement out your side into your pants, so they came up with a couple of more ingenious little devices call the "Flange" and the "Pouch". I remember saying to my mom that I could not imagine having something foreign attached to my body all the time. She would sarcastically say, "Aw son, it ain't so bad, you get used to it". Different companies make a variety of different flanges and pouches. There seems to be two different designs, one piece unit and a two piece unit. The first step to putting it on involves taking a template and measuring the diameter of your stoma. The flange has circles on the back representing different diameters. You then take scissors and cut the flange a little larger that your template size of your stoma. Everyone is different. You then peel the back of the flange off and fit it over the stoma and stick it to your body. The two piece design has a male ring on it. The pouch also has a ring on it that is female and they create a press fit that is waterproof. Most pouches are designed with an odor barrier so you cannot smell anything. The pouch can then be emptied and both are changed every so many days.

They had also removed a couple of polyps from my colon. Those are little things that grow from the colon wall. Polyps are most often benign (not cancer). But they did remove three of them and were going to biopsy them also. I would then find myself playing the waiting game again. I was watching a commercial one day about one of the Cancer Centers and the doctor said, "Cancer is the kind of diagnosis that makes you want answers now". Boy if that was not the truth! It was only a matter of days and I received phone call. They wanted me to schedule an appointment to come down to Indy and discuss the test results. It occurred to me on the drive down, that if my family medical history HAD been in the computer that day, my mother's history of Cancer may have never came to light and that tumor could have grown to stage four and killed me. Was this yet another coincidence? The meeting was in Indy and was with the head of Surgery so I was pretty sure I knew what that meant. I had Colorectal Cancer. A doctor and a couple of Interns from IU Medical came in for the meeting. He confirmed my suspicions although he told me I did not actually have Cancer yet. The tumor actually consisted of what are known as "High Dysplasia" cells, which always became Cancer. So for all intents and purposes, I had Cancer. The good news was that catching it so early greatly increased my chances of survival. Great news I thought.

This doctor was not the surgeon I was told, but he had met with them and the Oncologists (Cancer Doctors) and discussed my case. I basically had three options, one, do nothing and die of Colon Cancer someday. Not really an option I was thinking. Option number two was the permanent Colostomy I described before. The third option was what is known as resection. This is where they remove the cancerous portion of the colon and some extra for safe measure so to say, then they attach the two ends together and away you go. They felt that even though the tumor was very low in my colon, because of my age and activity levels, this was the option they were advising me to take. They said if it did not work out they could always do a Colostomy later. I do know that if I knew then what I know now, I would have had the Colostomy done from the very beginning after my first diagnosis. They then explained the risks that would be involved and problems that could occur. There was one warning that really caught both me and my wife's attention. They told me that where they would be operating would be right in the area of the main nerve bundle that controls the male sexual functions. They told me that they are obviously as careful as possible but sometimes things happen. They then told me there was the risk that I may never be able to have sex again. Man did my wife's eyes get big on that one. I knew I had a little time before I had to make the decision. We went home and discussed everything. We were really not too worried about not being able to have any more children, but no sex was another matter altogether. Even though they had said they would be careful, they made no promises. We were both still fairly young and the thought of no sex for the rest of our lives definitely had an effect on the decision making process. After a fair amount of research and discussion with a few friends that were doctors, we came to the decision that the resection was the best course of action. There were other treatments that I may have been able to get such as chemotherapy and radiation treatments, but I was fairly sure that would just be delaying the inevitable. I called the doctor the next day and scheduled the surgery. Little did I know at that time, but that would be the beginning of a nightmare that would last for almost the next ten years. As I said, if I had it all to do again, I would have had the Colostomy right then and saved myself a great deal of pain and suffering.

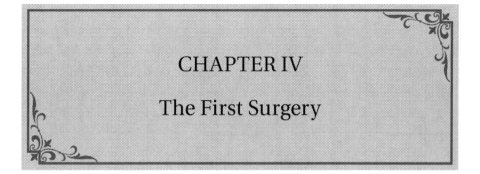

CHAPTER IV

The First Surgery

The surgery would be done at the Roudebush VA Hospital in Indianapolis. I was told that the doctor doing the surgery was a doctor from the Indiana University Medical Research Center. It is located next door and many doctors and interns do work for the Veteran's Administration. I thought that sounded promising. A medical research doctor had to be someone with a great deal of experience I figured. My wife and I went down to Indy the night before the surgery and again stayed at the same motel we had stayed at before. I was still pretty calm but I do know I said a great many prayers that night. The next morning we went to the hospital and I was admitted and prepared for surgery. I was asked if I had ever had an epidural. I said I did not even know what that was. They explained it was a form of anesthesia that was administered through the back into the spinal cord. I really do not remember why they wanted me to do it, but I did say yes. Something I have wondered about since then was whether it was a mistake or not. It may have been a contributing factor as to what was to follow and the problems I would have later. As the anesthesiologist was explaining everything I mentioned my previous experience and the vomiting. He said he would be able to give me something for that. The last thing I remember was counting backwards as they started to administer the anesthetic.

I woke up to find myself in the Recovery Area of the ICU. There was a nurse sitting next to me. I could not believe how good I felt. No pain or vomiting. I thought to myself this was a cake walk! I guess I was being way too active for the nurse's liking and he told me to settle down. I said I felt great and did not understand his concern. He told me it was only because the epidural had not worn off yet. Some time passed and I could feel the pain starting to creep in. It got worse and worse. It finally got to the point I could not take it anymore. It felt like someone had reached inside my abdomen and tore my guts out. He said I would be moved to my room momentarily and because this was Recovery, I could not get anything for the pain. He told me as soon as they got me to the room they would give me something for the pain. A short time later they moved me to my room and I was begging for something for the pain. They gave me some Oxycodone and a little machine I like to call a "Morphine Clicker". It is a little machine that has a hand held button and when you press the button, it pushes a little bit of Morphine into your IV tube. The only thing is, you only get so much and only every so often. Even though I had it and the Oxycodone, I was still in a great deal of pain. The pain was far worse than I had experienced with my neck surgery. My wife came in to see me and I told her I had never felt anything like this. I told her this was more painful than my car accident.

I did not see my wife for several days after that as we live about two hours northeast of Indy and she still had to work. Someone had to make some money and pay the bills. The next time she came she brought the kids. I was so glad to see them. They asked a lot of questions, but by the time they left, I think they were feeling better about things. They were now four and seven and they did not really understand what daddy had just been through or the pain I was in and I was surely not going to do anything to let them know. They just knew daddy looked ok now and was going to get all better. It was rather lonely. I had no visitors other than the wife and kids every so many days. The doctors and nurses came and went. Running their tests and checking my vitals and all the other things they do. Again I found out very quickly you will NOT get any sleep in the hospital. There always seems to be someone waking you up for some reason or another. After a few days the activity levels in my room seemed to increase. They were taking a lot more blood and I was starting to feel a little feverish. Then they started taking urine samples and just about anything else they could suck out of me.

It seemed as if I was starting to feel worse instead of better. The next morning the doctor came to visit and told me I had a fever. He told me they were starting to worry about an infection of some type. I was having what they called "swinging fevers". Up and down my temperature would go. My white blood cell count was also elevating quickly which is usually a sign of infection in the body. I was also a little embarrassed by the fact that I was wearing a diaper and could not control my bowels. I was told when I got there I would be there about five days or so. Well five days came and went and no one had said anything about going home. They said they were still concerned about the fevers and my white blood cell count. I was also starting to feel very sick and feverish. I was tired and fatigued and the pain was increasing dramatically again.

One morning they came in with a wheelchair and told me they were taking me to have a CT scan done. This is a high tech X-Ray that allows them to take pictures in slices and gives a great deal more detail for them to see. They asked me if I had ever had one before and I said I had not. They told me they would be doing this one with what they called "Contrast". They put an IV in you and push a radioactive dye into your system that makes the CT scan even better yet. After the test I returned to my room and found the dietician there waiting to see me. They wanted me to start trying to eat some food. Finally, real food I thought. It was mostly bland and soft but it at least helped to fill the void a little so I welcomed it anyways. The next day they said they wanted me to start trying to use the bathroom and try to have a bowel movement. The following morning I felt the urge and got up to go to the restroom. Moving at all was extremely painful and getting out of bed was almost unbearable. As I started across the floor I felt it. A total loss of control and whoosh, I felt my bowels let loose. It was running down my legs and forming a horrible smelling puddle in the middle of the floor around me. Here I was, a forty nine year old man standing in a puddle of diarrhea with it running down my legs wearing a dirty diaper. It was the ultimate humiliation. I do not think anything has ever embarrassed me since. They were doing a lot of testing and things were not getting any better. On the tenth day they decided to send me home. The doctor told me, "Sometimes these things take time to manifest themselves". I believe that is what is referred to as doctor speak.

The ride home was extremely painful. I felt every little bump that was in that road all the way home. If I had any brains I would have laid down in the back seat but I had been cooped up in that hospital for the last ten days and was ready to see a little of God's creation. We got home and I laid down on the love seat we had in our Family Room and proceeded to try and die. Every passing day I got worse and worse. By the time the ten days were up, I was so weak my wife and a neighbor had to load me into the car. My appointment was again with General Surgery in Indy. I had to wait for what seemed an eternity. I am sure a lot of that was my condition. Minutes seemed like hours. We were finally led into one of the examination rooms. A short time later, a doctor walked in. He took one look at me, his eyes widened, and he turned right around and left. He never said a word. A few moments later he returned with a nurse, a gurney and a woman from the lab. The doctor said I was septic or about to become septic and they were re-admitting me. So we headed up to ICU with a stop at the X-Ray department. They were going to do another CT scan. I got settled into my room and they started plugging in the IVs and pushing antibiotics and saline into me. A little later two doctors came into the room. One was the surgeon that had done my surgery. They told me that bacteria had leaked from my colon and had formed three abdominal abscesses. One between my bladder and colon, one on my lower right side and the last, and largest, along my colon where they had put the two sections back together. The one by the bladder was full of air and they were not too concerned about it. I was told the other two would have to be drained. This was to be the start of the ten year nightmare I mentioned before.

The next morning I was taken to Intervention Radiology. I was told they would be inserting drain tubes into the infected areas to drain the infection. Again I was amazed at the technology. They were looking inside my abdomen with an X-Ray machine that allowed them to see images in real time as they were sliding these drain tubes in so they would know exactly where to locate them. It was amazing. But again it was not without pain. First they administered a local anesthetic. Then they make a small incision to insert the tubes through. They are a vinyl looking tube with a small head on them. The head has holes in it for the infection to drain out through. The tube exits your body and runs to a collection bag that the infectious liquid collects in. When they are inserting the tube it is enclosed in what appeared to be a sheath of some type so they can control its direction. When it is located, they then open the sheath and pull it out leaving the tube inside you. Now comes the really fun part. They stitch the tubing to your side and every time you move it hurts. It is impossible to move without there being pain. Nothing great but damned annoying after you have them in for a few days.

The abscess on my lower right side was not that bad but the one along the colon on the other side was another story. It was huge and they drained over a liter of fluid about as green as your grass out of me in fifteen hours. I remember the nurse came in to empty the collection bag that evening and she dropped it and it spilled all over the floor. I do not think dead bodies smell that bad. The smell was so horrible I almost vomited all over her as she was cleaning it up. I was quickly getting to dislike hospitals. It seemed I was there for an eternity. They were trying several different antibiotics but nothing was working. After two weeks of battling the infection I was exhausted and my body hurt everywhere. I am not sure how many different types of antibiotics they tried but they finally seem to find the right one and I started to improve. After two weeks of IVs and this and that, I was ready to go home. The problem was I still was not urinating on my own. This was going to cause my stay to be extended. I prayed to God to help me. The next day a woman came in and said they would let me go home if I learned how to "Cath" myself. A Catheter is a tube they slide up the Urethral Tube of the penis to the valve in the bladder and forcing it open and causing the bladder to drain. You then remove the tube and dispose of it. You repeat this procedure every time you have to urinate.

Now I know you have heard all those macho sayings about how you are not a man until you can do this or that? Well I got news for you. You are not a man until you can "Cath" yourself. A few weeks passed and I was still in a lot of pain. The love seat in our family room was quickly becoming my home. It seemed if I propped my foot up on the back and turned a certain way, and took my pain medication, life was almost bearable. I was living on Oxycodone and fiber. They had me putting two tablespoons of fiber in water and drinking it twice a day. The fiber was causing my bowels to be loose and it burned my rectum horribly. When I would sit on the edge of the bed at night, it burned and hurt terribly. Bowel movements were becoming more and more painful. I was given all kinds of reasons why this was happening by the doctors, none of which turned out to be right in the end. I was quickly getting frustrated with life. I needed help and prayed more and more often. During this time I could see my kids were still worried. I did not interact with them much. The pain and frustration had taken over my life. I knew I was failing miserably as a parent. I should have been talking more with them and comforting them. Also, my marriage was starting to fail at this point. I was being a lousy dad and a lousy husband. I was consumed with my condition and the pain.

I finally said enough is enough and went to see the doctor. They ran another scan and discovered the source of all my pain and discomfort. Somehow, the tube they had inserted into the abscess along my colon had punctured the wall of my colon and was hanging inside. If it wasn't for bad luck, I would have no luck at all I thought. There was a problem though. They could not just pull the tube out or I would get feces leaking into my abdomen and I could be worse off than I already was and even die. I had to wait six weeks for a tube of flesh to form around the vinyl tube before they could remove it. Your body starts to reject the material the tube is made from and forms a flesh tube around the vinyl tube to protect your body from it. The first tube had already been removed from the other abscess by then and was no longer a factor. That abscess had closed off nicely and was no longer a factor. But this one was determined to break me. I was at wits end and ready to scream. Are you kidding me? Six more weeks of this thing stitch to my side, throbbing and hurting constantly. But wait it gets even better! As the flesh tube formed around the vinyl tube, watery feces and gas started to leak out my side. Nothing like pooping and farting out your side! My daughter made a few comments and even started to call me "Mr. Stinky". I was not hurt too much because I knew she did not really understand. I know they worried a lot.

The VA Hospital where we lived took a couple of X-Rays and sent them to Indy. They said it appeared it was time to pull the tube out. Thank God! So it was back to Intervention Radiology in Indy. I asked the doctors doing the procedure what would happen to the flesh tube after they pull the vinyl tube out. After all, I did not want this stuff coming out of my side the rest of my life. They told me the tube would collapse and the body would absorb the tissue. "Alright, but what about the hole left in my colon where you pull the tube out?" I asked. They said it SHOULD heal itself off. I then asked, "What happens if it doesn't?" He responded, "Then we will glue it shut". I thought he was joking but he was very serious. He informed me they glued tissue all the time. I had never heard of such a thing. I guess you learn something new every day. And you can believe me, I was quickly becoming a very learned individual about the field of medicine. They took the tube out two days before Christmas and I told my wife I was pretty sure it was the best Christmas present I had ever had. I thanked God for helping me get through this.

I spent the better part of three months laying on that love seat watching television and suffering. I prayed and prayed for God to heal me. I even made a promise to God that if he did, I would quit smoking and this and that. I did not keep my promises to God then and vowed I would never make another one to him because I knew I was too weak to keep it. Those types of promises always seem to come in times of desperation. Times when there seems to be no other way out except with the Lord's help. But as I said earlier, no wisdom yet. I thank God that he is forgiving and begged him for his forgiveness for my weakness. Breaking that promise has bothered me ever since and I have never forgot it. Soon they told me I needed to start walking and moving. I could not believe how much pain I was in when I tried to walk. It was winter outside in Indiana. I remember one evening going for a walk. I was wearing scrubs, a coat, hat and gloves. It was very cold and the snow was blowing straight sideways as I tried to venture down the side walk. I remember my neighbors looking out their front picture window at me shaking their heads. I cannot imagine what they were thinking. I was so amazed at how much you utilized your stomach muscles to walk. Again I was feeling that familiar feeling of great pain.

I spent the better part of that winter on that love seat. The doctor finally released me to go back to work after three months. It was at this point I also realized something else. I had been on Oxycodone for quite some time and had become addicted. I discovered this quite by accident when I thought I was going to run out of pain medicine and cut back to preserve the remaining doses for sleeping. I went into withdrawals. I shook and sweated for almost seven days. I went into it cold turkey. What a nightmare the next week was. I later told the doctor I had become addicted and he told me not to feel bad, that many surgery patients become addicted when on pain medication for as long as I had been. He then asked me what type of program I wanted to go into to break my addiction. I told him I was already off, that I just quit taking them and sweated it out. He was amazed at my self-discipline and said that no one ever does that. I told him I had some help from a little higher plane than ours. He must have been a spiritual man because he smiled and said, "Good for you".

CHAPTER V

Back to Work

After being given permission to go back to work, my first job was the largest and most physical I had ever had. I had to lay eighteen hundred square feet of sub-flooring, eighteen hundred square feet of ceramic tile (including eight bathrooms) and about a thousand square feet of heavy wood flooring. All this was on three different floors of a newly constructed home. I worked by myself with no help as I was always very leery about hiring anyone. People were just not as quality oriented as I was so I did all my jobs myself unless it was just unavoidable. I do not know how much you know about laying ceramic tile but it is not an easy job. Boxes of tile often weigh forty pounds or more. The bags of mortar are about sixty pounds each and the boxes of wood flooring were about seventy pounds each. The sub-flooring is four foot by four foot sheets of a material that is similar to thin drywall and also not light. One hundred twelve sheets of the stuff. All the sub-flooring is screwed into the floor. I had to put one hundred forty four screws in each sheet of sub-flooring. That's meant I had to bend over and screw in over sixteen thousand screws just to lay the sub-flooring. I think you are getting the picture.

Now imagine doing this after just having your abdomen cut open three months earlier. This job involves constantly stooping, bending and rising, not to mention the lifting and carrying of all this material up two or three flights of stairs to put it down. I would go to work in the morning with a pocket full of Percocet's to get me through the day. I remember the doctor later said in a follow up appointment, "Damn man, I told you that you could go back to work not build a house!" I guess he thought I worked in an office or something. He had never asked. At this point I was still experiencing a pretty fair amount of pain most of the time and bowel movements were still a problem. By this time, I was no longer seeing the surgeons and specialists but was again under the care of my regular doctor. I kept complaining about the pain and problems with bowel movements. Everyone I talked to kept telling me this should have passed by now. I tolerated it because I just thought that my job had probably extended the process with all the stooping and all. I told the doctor every time I sat down it felt like someone was shoving a cattle prod up my butt and pulling the trigger. She laughed.

More and more time passed and the pain was not subsiding. By this time she also was becoming concerned. She scheduled a wonderful test for me known as a Barium Enema. I began to think about the fact that no one had ever done any kind of a scan to find out if that hole in my colon where they pulled out the drain tube had actually healed itself shut. I soon found out. I went for the test and found that the technician that was assisting the doctor was one that had performed most of my CT scans. By this time he and I were old friends so to say. He explained the test would involve pumping a substance known as Barium through the rectum into my colon to see if there were any leaks. At that point there was an exchange a few humorous little tidbits I will not go into. Dave was a great guy with a sense of humor and we have come to know each other fairly well since then. The doctor came in and they started the procedure. They were behind me as I was spread eagle on a table with no pants on that was tilted forward a little. As I said before, humility is always a lesson that comes with medicine I think. They were looking at a scope of some type. The Barium works similar in this test as the "Contrast" dye I mentioned earlier works for the CT scan. They seemed to be looking and looking and finally the doctor said he could not see any leaks. About that time I had an itch and reached back to scratch. As I did, my torso turned a little and I suddenly heard this, "Whoa!"

from behind me. There WAS a hole in my colon and the Barium was pushing through. My body was trying to heal itself and had formed a flap of some type over the hole which would uncover when I twisted my torso. It had formed yet another abscess and a wonderful little thing called a fistula. A fistula is a little tube that the body forms to try and exit infection from an area.

I asked what could be done to fix the hole and the fistula. He mentioned a couple of possible options but said I would need to see yet another specialist to decide. I waited a long time for someone to call about it but no one ever did. I will say that I was my own worst enemy too because with all that was going on in my life at the time I did not press the issue. I would mention it to my doctor every time I went to see her. Years later, we found an entry in the computer that said she had referred me to Indy for a consult with some doctor there. That consult never happened and they and I both dropped the ball. I just kept living with the pain and discomfort and bowel problems. I was so concerned with work all the time. All the wrong things as they say. I wanted the bigger house for my family and all that. The materialistic behavior that seems to be so prevalent in our society today that is always at the expense of our ideals and families. Believe me folks it is just not worth it. When you lose your health your perspective of what is important in life suddenly changes very radically. I will say several times in this book. Once that time is gone, "IT IS GONE!"

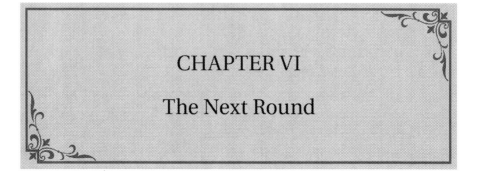

CHAPTER VI

The Next Round

By this time my marriage was becoming very shaky. I love my kids very much and was determined to stay married for their sake. Business was great though and I managed to keep my mind occupied with work. Again, I was not spending the time I should with my children. I knew that no one knew the pain and suffering I was experiencing though. I did not want to be a whiner and I did not want the kids to be worrying all the time. They seemed to have everything and were very much enjoying life, except I was not a very big part of that life. I became more and more distant from my family as my suffering continued. Yes I am an idiot for not doing something to change things. When you are in pain all the time and caught up in the rat race, your head seems to spin out of control. Judgment is not one of your better virtues at the time. I am sure a great many of you can relate. Things between my wife and I got worse and worse.

One afternoon, I was putting up a storm door and got some caulk on my finger. When I tried to flip it off I dislocated a tendon on my knuckle. Fortunately the job was done so I jumped into my truck and headed for the VA. They took an X-Ray and told me I had dislocated the tendon from the knuckle of my middle knuckle and put my hand and finger in a brace and told me to come back in two weeks for a follow-up. They told me it should re-attach itself but if it did not a minor surgery would be needed. Great more surgery I thought to myself. Two weeks later, I returned for the follow-up appointment but did not see my regular doctor. The doctor examined my wrist and told me it appeared the tendon had healed. As I sat there in her office I coughed. She looked at me and said, "That did not sound good". I told her I had smoked for forty years and everyone who smokes that long probably has some kind of a little hack.

She turned to look at the computer and then asked me if I had ever had a chest X-Ray since I had been in the VA system. I said that I did not think so. She asked me if I had time so I went up to Radiology for the X-Ray. She also said that she was going to schedule me for a consult with a pulmonary doctor. A couple of weeks later I was asked to come back for a CT scan. They did the scan and I went home. I guess I just did not connect the dots at the time. I came home from work one day and my wife told me there was a letter on the day desk from the VA. I looked at it and saw it was in the same envelope they always sent you when you have an appointment. I told her that it was probably my appointment with the pulmonary doctor. I did not pick up the envelope. The next day was a beautiful day and we decided to cook ribs on the grill. Dinner was great as everyone talked and enjoyed the great food. There was some pie on the counter so I got up to get a piece. As I went to get the pie I had to pass the day desk so I thought I would grab the letter and see when my appointment was. When I picked up the letter, it was thick and heavy and I could tell there was much more there than an appointment letter. I walked back to the table and sat down. My wife and kids were just finishing dinner.

I opened the envelope and inside was a form that the VA uses when they are sending you outside their system. I looked at the top of the form and it said "Procedure-Bone Biopsy". Now I was really confused, I thought there must be some kind of mistake. There were eight pages of material and on the last page it said, "Diagnosis". I quickly read what it said. I was shocked and horrified at what I read there. According to this form they were saying that the results of the CT scan they had run showed that they thought I had Bone Cancer, Liver Cancer, Lung Cancer, Thyroid Cancer and Lymphoma. I did not know what to say, what to do. And worst of all, I had read it out loud. The kids had heard me. How stupid could I have been to read it out loud in front of them? Silence struck the room. My mouth was hanging open and I was ready to cry. I looked at the kids and said this had to be some kind of a mistake that they should not worry. My kids went to bed and cried that night. There was hardly any response from my wife. I believe she was as shocked as I was.

I did not say it, but I knew that Lung Cancer and Liver Cancer were killers and if I really did have both, one or the other would probably kill me in two years or less. I am not really sure what I was thinking that night other than the feeling of sheer panic. I also know, I prayed to God more that night than any other night prior to that in my life. The next morning I called the VA to see what this was all about. They verified what the letter had said as being correct. I was in shock again. That evening the Chief of Surgery at our VA Hospital called and was falling all over herself with apologies and told me I was supposed to be called in and told by a counselor and an Oncologist. A little late for that I thought!

The bone biopsy procedure was at the same hospital I had my car accident in front of. The test was being done in the Radiology Department so up I went. They told me to undress and put on one of those little hospital diddys. You know the ones with the air conditioning in the rear. They led me into a room and I immediately recognized the CT scanner. The technician positioned me on the table and went behind the screen with the Radiologist and took a few slices with the scanner. The technician came back out and repositioned me and they took a few more. After they repeated this several times in different positions, I asked why all the repositioning? She then told me they were trying to figure out which angle would be the best to go in from. I did not understand and asked, "In where?" She said that once the found the best angle, they would be inserting a "Bone Gun" and taking a small piece of bone for a biopsy. Now I do not know about you, but the term "Bone Gun" in no way sounded like anything good to me. Finally she had me laid on my stomach. As I did my little gown fell open and my butt was exposed. She had a rather confused look on her face. Now I knew she had seen plenty of butts before and wondered why the look. She went back behind the wall and a moment later the actual Radiologist came out and looked at my lower back. He told me he could see a scar on my lower back and wondered how I got it. I told him it was where they took the piece of bone for the C-1/C-2 fusion I had done years earlier. He then told me that what they had seen on the CT scan was the spot where they had taken the piece of bone for the graft. He said the only anomalies in that area were the graft and my broken hip. I said, "Broken hip? I have never broken my hip". He told me it was plain as day on the scan. He said that it appeared to be maybe ten or twelve years old. Then it hit me..... the car accident! I had been immobilized and with all the other pain I must not have even felt it. I will say now that I am older I AM feeling it.

He then told me that what they thought may be a liver tumor was actually something called Hemangioma. That is a small ball of capillaries that had formed on the tip of my liver. Alright, two down, three to go I thought. He then said, "But now that thing in your lung is definitely a Cancerous Tumor and it is setting about a half an inch from your heart and I will not risk running a biopsy with it that close to your heart". He also said it looked like I had Thyroid Cancer. I am not really sure what it would take for me to have a nervous breakdown but I am sure I was stretched about as far I could be. A few days later I got another call. They wanted me to have something called a P.E.T. scan. This is yet another type of CT scan except instead of using dye to create contrast they use radioactive glucose. I was beginning to wonder how long before I would no longer require a flashlight to see in the dark. It seems that Cancer and infectious cells utilize glucose in a different way than normal cells. The radioactive glucose creates that great contrast they need to add more definition to what they are seeing. Cancerous cells appear as a brilliant light on the scan. When I got there they led me to a room that had a very comfortable recliner in it and told me to have a seat. A few minutes later, the nurse returned. She was wearing thick rubber gloves and was carrying what appeared to be a lead box with the red and yellow "Radioactive" symbol on it. She then opened the box and took out a syringe and inserted it into my arm and injected the glucose into me. She told me to make myself comfortable that we had to wait about an hour for the cells to absorb the glucose. After that they would do the scan. A full body P.E.T. scans. After the scan, I went home and worried and prayed. I think this is where God was really starting to teach me about faith. My life was just not going as planned.

A few days later I got a call from a friend of mine. I did not know it, but he was actually the Radiologist who was reading my scan. He was very straight forward with me as he knew that would be how I would want it. The tumor in my lung, the Thyroid Gland and some of the Lymph Nodes on the left side of my neck were all brightly lit. He told me he had done enough of these to know it was all Cancer. But as I had suspected he also said my pelvis and colon were also lit in such a fashion as to indicate some kind of serious infection there also. There WAS still something wrong down there. A couple of weeks later I had to return to the hospital for a biopsy of my Thyroid and Lymph Nodes in my neck. I had goiters on both sides of my neck that had been tested several years before and I was told they were Calcium deposits. I am so much more knowledgeable now. They had only tested the goiters the one time and many years had passed since then. I should have been pushing for periodical testing of them for more than just the reasons of Cancer. The biopsy came back positive for Papillary Thyroid Carcinoma. The lymph nodes had also tested positive for Cancer. So now I was faced with the fact that I had two new types of primary Cancer and a secondary type also. And I had already had the Colon Cancer the years before. Wow! How many types of Cancer can a guy get and still live I was wondering. As you can imagine I was filled with anxiety at this point. I did not figure my prospects were very good at this point. I was severely depressed. My biggest concern was my children. They were so young. Do I tell them or not? How do I tell them if I did? Too many questions and not enough answers. We decided not to tell them until we had all the facts about treatments and prospects for longevity of life and all.

I received a call from the head of Oncology at the Roudebush Hospital to come down and discuss my all my options. At the appointment, there was a discussion about the difficulty they were having finding a Thoracic Surgeon to perform the procedure on the tumor in my lung. Because of its proximity to my heart, no one wanted to do it. So they first had me meet with an Endocrinologist who specialized in thyroid and lymph node removal. He was young but seemed to be very knowledgeable of his field. He put a scope down through my nose and into my throat to look at my larynx and make sure everything was looking as it should on the inside of my throat. He then explained the procedure he would be performing on me. He would be making an incision from just behind the left ear down the side of my neck, across the base of my neck across the Thyroid and then part ways up the other side. He would then remove all of the Lymph Nodes on the left side of my neck and my Thyroid Gland. He would also inspect my Para-Thyroid gland to see whether it had been damaged by the Thyroid Cancer and also whatever Lymph Nodes he needed to on the right side. He was not sure how far up the right side he would have to go at this point because they had not tested the nodes on that side yet (Take note of this, it becomes a factor in the future).

This procedure they would be performing is known as a Modified Neck Dissection. I did not know what the Para-Thyroid Gland was so he explained it is a gland that sets behind the Thyroid Gland with four little tubes that run out and distribute Calcium to the body. I would first have the surgery to remove my Thyroid Gland. Then after a certain period of time, I would return to have a procedure where one day you take a radio-active isotope 123 in a capsule of iodine to illuminate the remaining Cancerous Thyroid Cells left in the body. Even though they would be removing the entire Thyroid Gland, a certain amount of particulate cells always remain and the isotope illuminates those cells. That is then followed up by another radio-active isotope 131 the following day that is supposed to kill those remaining cells. This just keeps getting better and better I thought. I was getting a heck of an education though. I remember trying to be clever and saying to him, "OK let me get this straight. You are going to slit my throat from ear to ear and I am going to live to tell about it?" He leaned over right next to my face and said, "Quite Literally!" I would end up with a three quarter smiley face under MY smiley face that looked a little like a cock-eyed grin.

Shortly after that I was contacted to make an appointment with a Thoracic Surgeon. He was from Serbia. He was working with the IU Medical Research Center next door and had agreed to do the surgery. Again I was relieved to discover that he was one of the top people in his field. A few days later we had a meeting. I really liked the man and he had a great bedside manner. He made me feel comfortable with what he was going to have to do. He would be performing a procedure known as a Lobectomy on my left lung. He would be removing the upper half of the left lung and then recommending a follow up of Chemotherapy as an added precaution. Lung Cancer is a killer he said. He was very up front with me which I respected and he did not say anything about the odds of success or any of that crap. He just said that quite often the Cancer is back within two years and quite often migrated up the Corotid Artery in the neck to the brain and formed a tumor there. He said the surgery would be performed using a method known as V.A.T.S. This is a video surgery that is minimally invasive. I also had severe Emphysema which was going to make the surgery even more difficult.

We scheduled the surgery for the first part of January. I then went and met with his technician for all the appropriate pre-surgery questions to provide any information he made need. I made sure to tell her about my previous bouts with Pneumonia and Empyema because I knew both of these had resulted in scarring that may affect what he was doing. I was now thinking about the fact that in the next year they wanted me to have half my left lung removed, chemotherapy, my neck slit and radioactive treatments. I was wondering who these people thought I was, Superman?

Again I found myself looking to God for help. These sorts of things make one look at life quite differently. I prayed for his help in getting me through all this and for help with my family. By this time it was just about a week before Thanksgiving. I was trying my best to get into the holiday spirit for the sake of the kids but found it extremely difficult to do. The first of January seemed to be just around the corner. Even though he had told me they would be using V.A.T.S. I was picturing many terrible scenarios in my mind. I was imagining everything from blood clots in the lungs to them having to get out the rib spreaders. I was sitting on the couch shortly before Thanksgiving thinking about my children and what kind of future they would have without a father, not that I was really being much of one anyways at this point. I was worried about the Cancer returning, wondering if I was on a long drawn out roller coaster ride to death. I had children from a previous marriage and had failed miserably as a father there and was determined not to do the same to these two. I was so angry at myself for still smoking. Prayer was becoming a very prominent part of my life now. I was on my knees begging the Lord for help. Asking that he keep his hand around me and give me the strength I needed to survive mentally and physically. Help me through this O' Lord I begged. My faith was growing as I started to think about a great many things at that time. Your perspective changes dramatically when face with death again and again as it seemed I had been.

CHAPTER VII

The Last Straw

About a week before Thanksgiving I was sitting on the couch in the family room contemplating what was to follow starting in five weeks. I was anxious and depressed. We had told the children and tried to explain all this to them in a way that we hoped would cause the least amount of anxiety for them. I do not think there is any way we could have said it that would not have devastated them. As I sat there looking at the television contemplating what was to come, my wife of twenty six years came in and sat down on the love seat. I could tell by the way she was looking at me and the way she was talking that she was leading up to something. I finally told her to say whatever it was she had to say. As you can imagine I was in no mood for much of any kind of conversation. She looked at me and said, "I want a divorce". Talk about kicking a man when he is down! But wait, it gets even better. Two days later, which was two days before Thanksgiving, she comes in again and says, "I just need for you to get out". I am pretty sure if I was ever going to contemplate suicide, it would have been that night. But as I said, I had become a much more spiritual person by this time. I had great faith in God by this time. I also pondered the story of JOB in the bible. I guess when my wife told the kids about the divorce, they let her have it with both barrels! So did many of her friends. The next day she came to me and said one of the stupidest things I think have ever heard come out of a person's mouth. She said, "Well, I guess you can stay until this Cancer thing is over". I do not want to spend time talking about the failure of my marriage but it helps you to understand how tough my situation was. The holidays came and went. I did at least get to enjoy Christmas with the kids. The birthday of Jesus set me to thinking and I was quickly starting to understand two things. One, I needed God to help me through this and I also needed something to live for. I knew that something was my children. "I cannot die! I have to children to raise" I said to myself. From that point forward, they became the driving force in my life that kept the earthly part of me going. The rest was up to God.

The first week of January arrived and down to Indy I went. My wife did stay for the surgery, but left shortly afterwards. I was under the knife for eleven hours again. The surgeon later told me later he wished I had told him about the Empyema because he had to spend two hours scraping scar tissue before he could even start the removal of the lung. I told him I had informed his technician during the interview with her. He informed me that most of the Emphysema on that lung was on the part he had removed and if I would quit smoking I could probably lead a fairly normal life. When I inspected the incision, I was surprised to see it was only about six inches long. He said that was the great thing about V.A.T.S. Minimally invasive! The drawback was the two big tubes coming out of the front and side of my chest for drainage. They were attached to places on the wall that said "Suction". They were drain tubes. And of course my old buddy Mr. Pain was back and working at full strength. He and I seemed to be becoming best buddies.

The Nurse came in and we talked about several things. I asked him how long before I could get up and start walking. He seemed a little surprised. I told him I wanted to start walking as soon as possible. I had learned from previous surgeries that you need to get moving as soon as possible. Doing so may be painful now but it is much more painful later if you do not and just prolongs the healing process. He looked at me and said, "You just had half your lung cut out man!" I told him that I did not care and asked if there was a medical reason why I could not. He told me he would talk to the doctor to find out when I could. Two days later he came in with a walker with a box on it. He showed me how to unhook the drain tubes from the wall and attached them to the portable box to drain into while I was walking. He also showed me how to re-attach them to the wall when I was done. He cautioned me and told me I would have to have a nurse unhook my IVs before I left though. He also told me to make sure to call when I got back to hook my IVs back up. Eventually, the IVs were no longer needed and I was able to come and go as I pleased.

He left and a short time later, I was doing laps around the nurses' station and up and down the hall and back again. The nurses were amazed. They could not believe I had a lobectomy two days before and was now walking up and down the hallway. I was determined not to let what happened after my colon resection happen again. A couple of days passed and I began to sense something was wrong. They started bringing medical students into my room to "View" me. I heard one of the students make a comment about something called "Subcutaneous Air". I was wondering what he was talking about. The next day the surgeon came in to see me. He then proceeded to tell me I had a hole in my lung from which air was leaking. That air then comes to the surface of the body and you start to blow up like a balloon, thus the students comment. I went to the mirror and was astounded when I saw my reflection. My God, I looked like the Stay Puff Marshmallow Man! He told me he wanted to wait a little while and see if a clot would form and seal off the hole. He said he believed the hole was somewhere along the seam they had formed where he had cut off the upper lobe of the lung. After a week, he returned to give me the bad news. They were going to have to open me back up, find the hole and seal it off. So here I was going back under the knife again! This was really getting to be a bad habit! The next morning he basically repeated the surgery he had just performed the week before.

Again I was doing laps around the nurses' station and up and down the hall. People were starting to make comments to me about how strong and determined I was and all that. I have never been able to take a compliment very well and usually cover my embarrassment with some kind of humor. I told them they were confusing strength and determination with stubbornness and stupidity. I just kept telling them, "By the grace of God, there go I". The doctor came in and emphasized his comment about quitting smoking again. I had not smoked for the two weeks I was there. The next morning they came in and removed the drain tubes. They kept pulling and pulling. I was shocked as they pulled them out to find they were almost nine or ten inches long. They had been inside my chest all this time. The scars they left were much more severe than the VATS scar was. I lost my morphine clicker about then too and was not very happy. By this time I was into the hospital routine, TV, food and walking consumed my day with a nap when I could.

A week or so passed and they came in and told me I would be going home the next day. I was so excited to be going home. The surgeon told me he was amazed at my ability to heal and how much strength of will I had. I told him, "Faith my friend, Faith in God". I also told him not to count his own skills as a surgeon out either. I knew it had not been easy for him either. Having known he had to deal with the Emphysema and the scarring from the Empyema. The fact that the tumor was located so close to the heart and the difficulties that must have presented. He thanked me for understanding his position and not being angry for about the need for the second surgery. I told him I was sure he had done the very best he possibly could.

I had only seen the kids once this entire time. When I got home I cried as they ran up to me and hugged me. I never wanted to let go of them. I missed them dearly. I little while later I asked my wife if she had started my truck while I was gone to charge the battery. She told me she had not so I got the keys and started it up. It started right up but I told her I was going for a drive to charge it anyways. It was just an excuse. It had been three weeks since I had a cigarette and I headed straight for the gas station and bought a pack. DO YOU BELIEVE THAT? What an idiot I was. Just had half my lung cut out I was still going to smoke. What was I thinking? My wife caught me and she was furious. I am not sure I had ever seen her so mad. But at the time I did not care, I believe my response was, "What do you care, you are divorcing me remember?" I was feeling so much stress and pain and I just used it to justify my continued smoking. My life was miserable. The kids were in school during the day and my wife locked herself in the study all day "working".

I was so selfish. I did not even consider the fact that her father had died from this horrible disease and here she was watching another love one waste his life away to tobacco. It must have devastated her. I was totally self-absorbed. They wanted me to wait a month for me to build my strength back up then we would start the Chemotherapy. They wanted to make sure my immune system could take it. My mother had been through Chemotherapy and I watched what it had done to her and was dreading the start of it. Later I would say that Chemotherapy was worse that the damn disease. I would not wish it on my worst enemy. I remember sitting in that chair for seven and a half hours every Tuesday for what seemed like an eternity while the ran five bags of stuff through me. They did lots and lots of blood draws to make sure the stuff was not killing me. They were checking to see if it was killing off my bone marrow and my white blood cells, essentially killing my immune system. The very first time I did it I never even made it home before we were back at the hospital. My stomach was producing HUGE amounts of stomach acid and my guts were on fire. They wanted to admit me but I said I had spent enough time in hospitals lately. They gave a very strong proton pump inhibitor and I was drinking half a bottle of Maalox Plus a day to deal with it and lying in pain and suffering as my children watched and cried. It was horrible.

I did try to do a small job to get out of the house and get some exercise. The money was desperately needed too. It was only putting up a storm door. This was a job that was usually fairly easy and did not take very long to do. It took me all day. I was exhausted and hardly able to breathe by the end. I thought I was going to die. So now it appeared I could not work. My wife was not really working then. She had a "Job", but it was basically a part time thing that did not really pay much. I had never asked her to work because I did not want the children growing up as "Latch Key" kids. She could spend the time needed with the kids and do the parenting needed during the day. This is where the financial portion of our lives began to collapse. I was soon becoming concerned about losing our house. We were getting further and further behind. Then out of the blue, one of my family members called and told me they were going to pay our bills. They were concerned that all the stress about finances would hinder my healing. I cried. That is actually a somewhat vague description of the way it happened because all family members acted anonymously at the time and swore me to secrecy.

I will say this to all of you. If you have a loved one or family member that has Cancer, extend every bit of financial aid you can to them. My health care was free and we were still going broke. I cannot imagine what medical bills associated with Cancer would be in addition to the burden I was already experiencing. I will never be able to repay my family for the help they extended me during this time and I will mention the fact that my family members are not wealthy people. This whole ordeal has created friction between them and I but I still love them dearly for all their help. My family and I would have been destitute if it was not for them. The months seemed to drag on and on. I was lying around feeling miserable all the time. Worrying about what was to come. Again I was neglecting my children. I was so selfish and self-absorbed. Hurting or not, I still had a responsibility to be a parent. It does not take much effort to just talk to them. They told me later they were sad for me and stayed away because it was hurting them to see me in pain all the time. After all, they were only ten and seven by this time. My illness was so much a part of their growing up. I was a source of much sadness at a time when they should be enjoying life to the fullest. They should have been happy children with all the wonders that accompany growing up. It often makes me cry to think of what they have been through.

The problem was, it was not over yet. Finally the Chemotherapy was over and I was thanking God for helping me through it. Never again I thought, never again referring the Chemotherapy. It was at this time I was also beginning to wonder just what God had in store for me. It was quickly becoming obvious that I was one of those individuals that he makes a little extra effort to protect from themselves and the perils of life. I could not understand it considering my past. It was becoming obvious that there was something he wanted me to do.

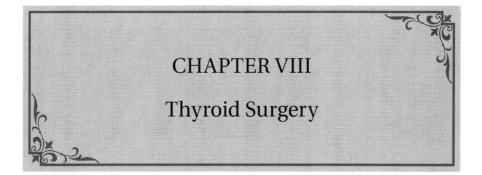

CHAPTER VIII

Thyroid Surgery

They waited a month for my body to recover from the Chemotherapy and get strong enough to withstand the next surgery. Yes, a whole month. I was still in that negative frame of mind I had been for some time now. I prayed and hoped. I was still experiencing a great deal of anxiety over finances also. My family was helping but it was a matter of time before that would end. As I said, they were not wealthy people. The day came for the Thyroid Surgery and as before, we went down the night before as the surgery was early the next morning. Why is surgery always at zero dark thirty? Don't surgeons ever sleep? My wife's brother came up to be with her during the surgery. The surgery was another long one. Apparently they brought me out of the operating room and had not cleaned me up yet and wheeled me right past my wife and her brother. You could see the thirty some staples in my neck and all the blood. Lots of blood she said later. She told me when her brother saw me, he almost fainted. I woke up feeling the pain but by they had already set up my Morphine Clicker and I knew just what to do with it. The nurse came in with some Oxycodone also and that helped. The next day the surgeon came in to see how I was doing. The Thyroid Gland converts iodine in our bodies which we get mostly from the salt we eat into a hormone that almost every organ in the body utilizes in some way, shape or form. It is the key gland to controlling our metabolism. Since I no longer had a Thyroid Gland, I would now be dependent on a synthetic form of the hormone called "Synthroid" for the rest of my life. Something I was not thrilled about. Not having the drug for a long period of time would eventually kill me.

Finding the correct dosage can be very tricky too and take considerable time. He also explained that my Para-Thyroid was basically destroyed also and that I only had one of the four tubes left. He had tried to reconstruct one of the others but did not know how successful that would turn out. He also had to relocate a main saliva gland that would turn out to be the source of much pain also creating a condition known as "First Bite Syndrome". Every time I would eat for the next several years, when I took the first bite of food and began to chew, my jaw would burn badly. I also had two drain tubes coming out of my neck. They love them drain tubes I thought. I had a fourteen inch long incision in my neck and thirty two staples holding it all together. You cannot imagine the discomfort. I am not talking about the pain. This was something else altogether. For almost a month, it felt like someone had their hands on my throat choking me all the time and it was extremely hard to swallow as you can imagine.

I woke up and was in the recovery room. They wheeled me up to the ICU and as we entered the ward all the nurses started saying things like, "Hey, Bill's back" and the like. Now you know you have spent way too much time in ICU when the nurses all know you by your first name. The good part was, they all knew me and I knew them which led to excellent treatment. They all knew if I pressed that nurses' button, it was for a damn good reason and they always responded quickly. The Roudebush VA hospital has a great ICU and a great staff running it. They are all to be commended for their caring and professionalism. I was beginning to notice the astonishment of the doctors and nurses at my ability to persevere. I do now, and always will, attribute that to God. As I said before, by this time I understood that this was not me but the Lord who wanted me to survive. I am just a human being like everyone else. It is him, not me, who is responsible. And I always made the standard reply when anyone said anything. "Not me, it's the Big Guy upstairs".

A week or so went by and they told me I would be going home in a couple of days. I was very excited to get home and see the kids. My wife had not brought them down this time and I missed them dearly, but previous experience had taught me not to get my hopes up until I was on my way out the door. And I soon found out my thinking was justified. Surprise, there was a problem! I was still draining too much fluid through the drains in my neck and could not go home until the amount of drainage dropped to a certain amount. That took three more days. I finally went home. This time going home was different. I was feeling some of the fight in my spirit starting to die. I was exhausted and anxiety was setting in again and taking its toll. I was easily irritated and was angered by the most trivial of things. The choking feeling was not helping either. I finally got to the point of frustration that I almost tried to pull out the staples with a pair of pliers. It was time to pray again. I rarely asked God for things for myself, but this was one of the times I did. I needed his help and I knew it. The table next to the love seat looked like a pharmacy. I was also giving a great deal of thought to my marriage and wondering when the end would come. The kids were horrified at the sight of my neck and stayed away. I think it was hurting them more than it was me. By this time my wife and I had not slept in the same bed for quite some time. I would lie in bed at night and sob, praying my children did not hear me in the adjacent bedrooms.

When you have Cancer, there is always a thought in the back of your mind as to whether it will ever come back. Today we know so much more about this horrible disease than we did then. Even in the few years that have passed since then, great strides have been made in genome research that I believe will eventually lead to the cure for a great many diseases. But until we do, many people will suffer and many people will die. I see commercials on television for the St. Judes Children's Hospital on television and I cry. I am an adult and know what I have been through. I cannot imagine what a child must feel or their parents when they are diagnosed with Cancer. And the thing was, every time I went to Indianapolis to the VA Hospital there, I drove right past it. I know one thing. If I ever win the lottery that hospital is going to get a very large check! At this point I was making a lot of trips back and forth to Indy. Follow ups on the surgery to remove the staples and a number of tests to monitor a great many things. I was also told what I needed to do to get ready for the upcoming radioactive isotope tests I mentioned earlier. As I said the body converts the iodine in the salt we eat into the hormone we need for metabolism. I was astonished to discover how much salt is in the foods we eat. It is one of the main preservatives in our foods. I got an education in nutrition during this time. I had to go on a special diet for a period of time before they could perform the procedures. I was allowed one hundred fifty milligrams of salt a day and four ounces of meat. To put that in reference, a slice of bread contains one hundred forty milligrams. I found out that one of the frozen dinners I ate regularly contained one thousand two hundred and fifty milligrams!

So, this is how this works. Thyroid cells search for iodine in the blood and consume it. By depriving yourself of the salt, they almost become like a junkie looking for a fix. The first isotope is put in a capsule of iodine and when consumed, those cells suck it up. This isotope is then scanned and any of those cells show up as bright light on the scan. The next day you return to take the other isotope in another capsule of iodine and that isotope is supposed to kill any of the remaining Thyroid cells in the body. As I said before, man's ingenuity never ceases to amaze me. After you finish this test you are not able to get within six feet of anyone because yes.... you are radioactive. You flush the toilet three times and wash the shower out and a few other things after using them. Thanksgiving was a few days away and my wife came to me and told me it was time for me to move out. On Thanksgiving Day I knew I truly did have something to be thankful to God for, my Life!

CHAPTER IX

Loneliness, Depression and Despair

My brother was also recently divorced and owned a house in the same subdivision as mine. He extended an offer to me to move in with him and his son. It was very kind of him to do so, but some of his conditions kept me from saying yes. I soon found a two bedroom apartment and started back to work again. Right before my earlier lobectomy, I had been fortunate to get a commercial tile job and had put all the money away in anticipation of the moving out. I knew I would need a pretty fair amount to make a new start. I will point out that at this point I was still experiencing a great deal of pain in my lower abdomen and having problems with bowel movements as a result of the earlier colon resection. I had been contacted by a new builder. The only problem was, he was way behind in the completion of these new homes and was needing the tile work completed as quickly as possible as it was one of the few steps that needed to be done before they closed on these homes. I was still experiencing the problems I had before with my bowels, not to mention that pain was becoming a permanent part of my life, but I was anxious to get started because the money was good and it would help alleviate some of my financial problems.

They pushed me hard to get the houses completed so they could close on them. It was also about this time my breathing was becoming a huge issue in my life and I was diagnosed with C.O.P.D. (Chronic Obstructive Pulmonary Disease). In my case, it was the Emphysema and it was only getting worse because I had still not quit smoking. The VA gave me a wonderful device called a Nebulizer. It is a little compressor with tubing and an attachment that takes small amounts of medicine and atomizes it into a steam like mist that you inhale and it opens the bronchial tubes. I was also now on a steroid I would inhale twice a day. If you did both medications properly at the same time, you felt pretty good for a while.

I was working long and hard hours to get these houses completed for closing. This was not good as I was quickly running myself down and getting sicker and sicker. It became very difficult but I kept pushing. I would get home at night exhausted and wanting a shower. It was a dirty job and I always felt so much better after a hot shower. That had all changed. I now dreaded showering as the hot humid air made it difficult to breathe with my COPD. My lungs would fill with mucus and I would start to panic as it became more and more difficult to breathe. Suffocating is a horrible experience and at this point, it was becoming a very familiar part of my life constantly. Suddenly my health started to deteriorate very rapidly and very dramatically. The work was very physical and my breathing problems seemed to be getting worse and worse. The work was in houses that did not have water on in them yet, and tile takes a lot of water. I was carrying two five gallons buckets at a time from houses across the street over rough ground and through the snow. It was winter and the air was cold and all this was exhausting me. I was working with sixty pound bags of mortar and grout. When I think back, this was one of the most trying times of my life. I was sick but I had bills to pay which now included Child Support. I was almost finished with the last house when they notified me that they were concerned about my health and this would be the last house I would be doing for them.

Bowel movements were becoming all but impossible. I was no longer seeing my children daily and it was killing me emotionally. They were the only thing keeping me going and now I had lost the daily love and joy I used to get from them. I also found out there was little financial help for people with Cancer. There was tons of money for research but try to get help paying the bills. Money was going out faster than it was coming in and I was panicking again. A couple of family members were still doing what they could but it was becoming increasingly difficult to fend off creditors and pay my every day expenses. My family had already done so much for me and it was creating a great deal of friction between some of them and me. I had been to the doctor's several times with my problems but since I was never running a fever, the urgency was just not there. This had been going on for almost two years now and had me frustrated to no end.

One day I went to work and could not even get half way through the day. I seemed to have so many problems and no solutions. It all seemed to run together after a while. After a weekend of pain and suffering I went to the Emergency Room at the VA Hospital on Monday. I told the doctor I recognized these symptoms, I knew it was another abscess. My doctor said she doubted it since I did not have a fever. I became angry and after some discussion she agreed to schedule a CT scan and I went up to the lab for blood work. She told me to go home and get some rest and she would call me the next day to let me know when the CT scan would be. My white blood cell count was extremely elevated so that indicated something was very wrong. I stayed home from work the next day as I felt so bad. When I stay home from work you know something is VERY wrong. The following day was Wednesday and I had to try and get some work done. I did not make it even half way through the day. I was no longer able to move my bowels so I stopped on the way home to get a bottle of the prep they give you for Colonoscopies. It emptied me out but I was immediately clogged by the next day. I found out when I was to receive the CT scan I was fit to be tied. It was TWO WEEKS away. I would be dead by then I thought. I tried to finish the job the next day but could not. One of the things I had never thought about when I moved out was a thermometer. So I stopped and got one on the way home. It read 103.

Friday when I returned to the VA Emergency Room with a fever and low and behold, I could now get my CT scan done stat (right now)! As I had suspected, I had not one but two abscesses. My doctor was so embarrassed. I am happy to say, she is no longer with the VA. One of them was an enormous pelvic abscess. It was under so much pressure, the infection sac had formed a knob that was protruding through my left buttock muscle. I think they were starting to panic about then for fear it would burst and fill my abdomen with infection. I quickly found myself being loaded into the back of an ambulance and on my way to a hospital located just up the block. The VA Hospital in my town was not staffed or equipped to handle this type of emergency at that time. When I arrived at the other hospital, they threw me into a room that had been converted from an office to an examination room and just left me there. I had heard stories of bad things happening to people who were transferred from VA Hospitals to public hospitals. There seemed to be some kind of class warfare going on here. They did at least come in and hook up an IV to me. I laid there for what seemed like the longest time. I was in some of the most severe pain I had ever felt, and as you know, I knew what severe pain was.

I finally had to go to the restroom and called to a nurse as she was passing by. She unhooked my IV and pointed to the bathroom. She never even bothered to come back and hook my IV back up. How rude I thought. Finally one of the ER doctors came into the room and said they had finally managed to get my CT scan downloaded and he was waiting for a Gastrointestinal Surgeon to get there. Right at that very moment the surgeon walked around the corner. They walked off together to go look at my CT scan. The surgeon walked back in a few minutes later shaking his head as he entered the room. The first thing he said was, "That thing has GOT to hurt! REALLY BAD"! His jaw fell open when I told him I had been working laying tile until the day before. He made a comment about giving new meaning to the term "Tough as Nails". He then told me I had some kind of Pelvic abscess that I can no longer remember the name of and that as soon as an Anesthesiologist got there, they would be operating.

By this time I was joking about becoming a doctor with all this knowledge I was acquiring about all these different systems of the body. He came over to me and said, "Let me show you something".

He put my finger on the knob protruding from my left buttock and I gasped. How had I not felt this before while bathing or something? Soon the other doctor arrived and they got started. As I came to, I was gasping for air. I could not breathe and was panicking. They had a breather ready for me and started to get me breathing again. The nurses could see the panic in my eyes. As I have said, suffocation is one of the most horrible things you never want to experience. I always said the worst way to die would be to burn to death. The next would be to suffocate. I now had a hole in my buttock that went from my colon through the fistula and out my buttock muscle and exited the body. That now meant that any liquid feces that exited my colon would run right out into my pants. This also meant it was back to diapers again. He said he was then going to refer me back to the VA but said that he felt the next step would probably be an Ileostomy.

Believe it or not, after a couple of days in the hospital, I was back to work again. That job I had started was not finished and I was again going into panic mode about finances and needed the money. I had this delusion at that time I would someday be able to return to work as a normal person. I would go to work in my diaper and by the time I got home, my diaper was full of feces and I stunk horribly. Thank God my customers were so understanding. I cannot say enough about how low I was at this point. Can you imagine going to work and working in a diaper full of feces all day? I was exhausted and humiliated. I was soon finished with the job. I would start new jobs and this whole ordeal went on for weeks. I looked up and asked the Lord for his help again. I now look back and realize this was the ultimate lesson about pride and humility. Business was soon going south as quickly as my health as people were not spending due to the financial crisis created by the collapse of the housing market a couple of years before.

Again I found myself having to rely on my family for help. I was so embarrassed. I soon found myself unable to pay my rent, my creditors or anything other than food pretty quickly. I was destitute. My brother had been dating a woman and they had decided to get married. They bought a home in a small town north of ours. He told me I could move into the old house with my nephew until they got ready to sell it. The good part was, my children were now about a thousand feet away and I would be able to see them almost daily if I wanted. The night I moved into my brother's, my daughter came over to see me. She looked at me and told me I looked very bad and should go to the hospital. Later that evening I started to feel sick and vomited. I knew something was really wrong. I went to the hospital. I was septic. My blood filled was filled with infection and poison. They immediately transferred me to a brand new hospital on the north side of town. I was immediately started on antibiotics and saline. They were even talking about a blood transfusion. My veins were becoming more and more difficult to get IVs started into because of the Chemotherapy I had received earlier. It makes the veins hard and brittle. Once an IV is started it is difficult to keep it in for long as the vein then explodes easily under pressure.

I was extremely ill and I knew it. This was life and death kind of ill. A couple of days later I heard a couple of doctors standing outside my room discussing my case. I heard the one doctor say, "If we don't get a handle on this guy by tomorrow, he is going to die". I do not know if he did not think I could hear him or what but I yelled out the door, "Hey Doc, I can hear you!" They moved down the hall out of range of my hearing. They were doing a lot of other tests I had never had before. They even brought in a doctor that specialized in infectious diseases. Now that got my attention. I never did hear what she had to say about what was going on. Prayer was becoming a very large part of my life by this point. The next day two technicians came in and ran an ultrasound on the right side of my neck. They took lots of pictures and I knew from the discussion they had found something. They would not tell me what it was but I had a pretty good idea. It did not take much to put two and two together. They had found a lymph node that contained what they suspected was Cancer. It was very small and non-aggressive I was told later. They told me to talk to my Oncologist when I returned to the VA. It was becoming more and more difficult to continue with this new diagnosis. About that moment, when I was thinking

I could go no lower, again, my son and daughter walked in with big smiles on their faces and ran to give me hugs and kisses. I told myself, THEY are what you have to live for! They are too young and need a father. I prayed and reached as far down inside myself as I could for more strength. My prayers were answered and I slowly started to recover and my blood cleared. Two weeks later I was on my way home.

I spent most of the winter in and out of the hospital though. Infection had taken over my lower abdomen and my immune system was being overloaded again and again. I was so lonely, so depressed as I would lay in my bedroom day in and day out. Smoking cigarettes and watching television. I felt I was on a fast track to death and helpless to do anything about it. Most of my family lives in Alabama and a sister in California. No emotional support at all except for the visits I would make to see my kids. I would put on my coat and walk through the cold winter air and snow all hunched over looking like death warmed over. My kids seemed horrified by my appearance most of the time. They were a mixture of emotion. Going to see them at their (My) house made it hard too. The contrast of remembering all those wonderful times spent in that house and comparing them to the present. Again I must say if anyone was ever a candidate for suicide, I sure was at this point.

I knew that God was keeping me alive though for some reason I could not fathom. They say God uses adversity to build strength and character. I was convinced that whatever it was he wanted me to do, it must be a real doozy considering what I had been through. Actually I have never blamed God for my misfortunes when it came to my health. I always do just the opposite. I have always blamed Satan for all the misery on this earth. He had dangled all of life's temptations in front of me, and most of my life I had very eagerly grabbed ahold of them. I had no one to blame but myself. I was called into the VA a few days later. One of the recent scans had convinced them that if something was not done soon I was going to die. My abdomen was so full of infection it was inevitable. After much discussion it was decided that I would return to Indianapolis to see a specialist there and be evaluated to see what the best course of action would be. If you are reading this and are not a spiritual person, I want you to think how I am possibly alive at this point if not by the Grace of God. Think about it.

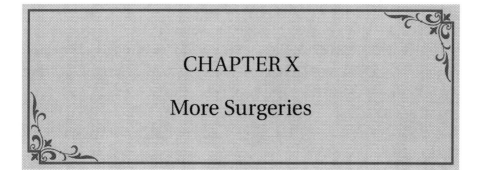

CHAPTER X

More Surgeries

I then went back to Indy to meet with a Gastrointestinal Specialist and surgeon. He had quite a reputation amongst the staff there and so again I was hopeful. Never lose hope or you are dead. He told me that he wanted to perform a surgery that would stop the flow of feces through the fistula and reroute it back though my rectum again. He warned me that this would take some time and possibly more than one surgery to accomplish. I did not care I was ready to try anything. There was only one problem, I would have to wait six weeks for the surgery due to the backlog in patients waiting for surgery in his department. I was thinking a lot about God and my future. I think it was at this point I was starting to try more than just the traditional prayers. Experimenting to make a spiritual connection with God in ways I had never heard of people trying before. My views of him became much more spiritual instead of the earthly words and images I was used to. One thing was very apparent to me at this point, I was still alive at a time when almost every doctor I met said most would have given up. My perspective of life was changing. I was beginning to understand that it is not our time here that is important, but what comes after. Finally it was time for the surgery. It was getting close to Christmas again. The doctor said it would be a little while after the surgery before we would really know the results. As you can imagine, I was pretty down at this point with Christmas near but managed to keep pushing myself. I thought of my kids and their smiles and knew I just could not pass until my job with them was done. As I have said over and over again, "By the Grace of God there go I". I was now seeing that whether or not I understood why, I had made some kind of a connection with God that most probably never find. This enabled me to find the fortitude I needed to keep going. He helped me reach down deep inside myself and find that genetic desire to live that I spoke of at the beginning of this book.

Christmas Eve arrived and no one had come to visit since I had been in the hospital and I was very depressed. Then surprisingly, a nurse came in and said they were going to release me. I was ecstatic for a moment. Then it suddenly occurred to me, I had no way home. It was late in the day and the D.A.V. van had already left for my town so that was no longer an option. I also knew many people had already left for the holiday and that would probably make my discharge take even longer. The place was like a ghost town. As much as I did not want to, I needed to bite my tongue, swallow my pride and work up the courage to call my brother and ask him to come get me. That would mean a three hour round trip and it was five o'clock in the evening now, we would not get home until eight that evening. He did reluctantly come after me. He will never understand how much it meant to me at the time. I would now be home for Christmas with my kids that I had not seen for over a week. We hardly spoke on the way home. I could barely sit as my rectum hurt so badly from the surgery. He dropped me off at the house and went home.

The next day was Christmas and he invited me and my kids to Christmas dinner. It was strange how much I was learning to appreciate the truly simple things in life again such as family and food. I did not think my brother was all that spiritual a person so I thanked God in my own mind for letting me be there with them all. I have a picture in front of me on my coffee table that was taken that day. I will always treasure it. It is funny how daughters capture a special place in their daddy's hearts and it is still that way today. That was almost seven years ago now. It seems like an eternity ago. I went back to my brother's old house after dinner. The days seemed to drag on as I prayed for improvement in my condition. After several weeks

I returned to Indy for an examination with the surgeon. Much to my disappointment, he did not see the results he had hoped for. He said he was going to have to do yet another surgery. He said he needed to remove more tissue than he had originally thought. I think the ICU nurses thought I was looking for a job there. A couple of days later, it was time for the other surgery.

They put me under but I woke not all that long after I went under only to find that he had come to the conclusion now, that I was going to need a permanent colostomy. As you can imagine, I was very disappointed. I knew that it meant I would have to have a least two more surgeries. The first would be an Ileostomy. That is where they separate the small and large intestine so that the colon, or large intestine, can drain of any food and infection before the permanent colostomy can be performed. A few days later they performed the Ileostomy. I remember waking after the surgery to find a little piece of my intestine protruding from my side. It was so odd to see it sticking out my side. A piece of my guts coming out my side, wow! Then the Ostomy nurse came in to give me instructions on how to put the flange and pouch on. She told me what foods not to eat as they may cause blockages and so on. She warned me that I must be prepared for accidents. There will be accidents and most of the time they will be very embarrassing. My mind immediately went back to that day after my resection when I was standing in the middle of the floor in a diaper surrounded by diarrhea and I was thinking, "I doubt it". I had always been in excellent shape for my age and was now seeing myself as more and more broken. I was now dependent on man and his pills and gadgets to survive. It was quite a humbling experience. I was obviously not a quitter, but God had to come and give me another dose of fight at this point. The fight I would need to get back on my feet and get going again. A few days later I was allowed to go home. The ride home was the usual painful bumpy ride. My brother dropped me off at the house and went home.

My mental state was not good and I found myself deeply depressed again and all alone. I wondered how much a man truly could take before he did something stupid. Time for prayer I thought. I knew somehow he was there watching me and taking care of me. How could he not be, I am still here. It is a strange sense of confidence that accompanies faith. I calmed down and concentrated on putting myself into a better frame of mind through prayers. I am sure that most people around me had little knowledge of the spirituality I was developing. The infection had pretty much taken over my lower body at this point. Showering had become an enormous task. The infection was also exasperating my respiratory problems. I had to make several trips to the VA Emergency Room to deal with these attacks. One night I woke up and was soaked. My pouch had broken open and the couch and I were soaked with runny feces. I was alone and had to clean it up and it was exhausting. I guess she was right, accidents will happen. I was hoping this was not a sign of things to come.

My coughing continued and I guess the severe contracting of the stomach muscles had caused my stoma to break loose from my abdomen. My intestines were pushing out and into my pouch. This made putting the flange over it extremely difficult. The coughing worsened and I ended up back in the hospital. One night I needed to change my pouch and take a shower so the nurse accompanied me to the shower. She stood outside while I showered. As I removed my pouch, much to my surprise, my small intestine had pushed almost two feet out of my abdomen. I could not get it to go back in so I called to the nurse. As she was an RN, I guess I thought she would know what to do. I will never forget the look on her face as she pulled the curtain aside to see me standing there holding two feet of my small intestine in my hands. She was flabbergasted. Her eyes were as big as silver dollars. Well as it turned out, she had no idea what to do and ran off to get the doctor. This meant I would be going back to the Operating Room for a little fix it surgery. Part of the problem was that I was having to wait to have my colostomy because of the backlog of patients. I have my own ideas as to why, but the Oncologists I had spoken to were amazed at the number of Cancer cases coming out of Northeast Indiana.

I knew I was slowly dying and if something was not done soon, all the infection in my lower abdomen was going to kill me. I felt myself slowly fading day by day. I was staying at my brother's still. He had been talking to my sister in Alabama. She and my parents lived just outside of Birmingham. My brother wanted to sell the house and everyone had just about had their fill of Bill and his health problems. My brother called me one morning and said we needed to talk. He and his wife came over a little later. After many questions, I began to realize this was about getting me out of the house so they could sell it. They also seemed angry about something. I was a bit confused because my brother had told me they wanted to do several things to the house before they sold it, and since I was a contractor, he wanted me to supervise. Now he seemed angry and told me he had been on the phone to my sister in Alabama. I was now within three weeks of my scheduled Colostomy surgery in Indy. As I sat there, he told me that the following day he would be driving me down to meet my sister half way and she would pick me up and take me to their house. They had talked to the Birmingham VA and made arrangements for me to set up the surgery there. I did not know what to say. Considering my predicament, I was at their mercy and did not have any choice. I was dying and destitute. I was receiving another lesson in pride and humility. I really had no alternative so the next morning I got into the car and we left.

Again, there was not much conversation. He appeared to be angry and I knew any discussion would just make matters worse. I did not understand what he was angry about. Well apparently he had changed his mind about me supervising the work and I was now on my way to Alabama. My sister met us as planned and we headed for Birmingham. My sister then told me her husband was not too happy about me staying with them so I would be staying with my parents instead. At least I would be able to spend some time with my mother as I did not get to see her often because of them living so far away and her health. When we arrived at my parents everyone was shocked at my appearance. They had no idea I looked as bad as I did. I am not a large man, but I had always been pretty muscular and that was the man they were used to seeing. Since they never saw me, the contrast between the old me and the new me was rather shocking. Before all this started I weighed about one hundred fifty five pounds and as I said was in good shape. I now weighed about one hundred twenty two pounds and was thin and white as a ghost. The next day I called the VA in Birmingham and made an appointment. I was able to get in very quickly and get an appointment for the following week to be assigned a primary care doctor and discuss the surgery. When we arrived, I was pleasantly surprised to find that it was a very well staffed hospital.

The University of Alabama at Birmingham has a medical program and it seems they have a relationship much like Indy had with the IU Medical Research Center so there were plenty of doctors and interns around. I met with my doctor. She walked in and we made the usual introductions and she sat down to pull up my medical history on the computer. She kept looking at the computer and then at me. She did this several times before I finally asked her if something was wrong. She said she could not believe how good I looked considering what she was reading. She said she could not believe I was even still alive. She even made a comment that if someone who looked as good as me had told her that what she was reading on her screen had happened to them, she would call them a liar. I told her God loved me and had held me tight through it all or I would not be here. She could not believe my demeanor. I told her I would never lose my sense of humor no matter what. She then scheduled an appointment for me with the surgeon that I would need to see about getting my Colostomy done.

A week later I arrived for my appointment with the surgeon. As I walked in, I could not believe my eyes, she was nine months pregnant and due any day! I would have to wait for her to have the baby and come back from maternity leave. I could have had my surgery done by then if I was back in Indiana. She saw my condition and immediately started me on a regiment of antibiotics. Care had to be taken to make sure this did not present any complications for the surgery. I left feeling as if I was taking one step forward and two steps back. I was not feeling too good though as here I was, a fifty year old man living with his parents, dependent on others for everything from my health to my food. This was such a total contrast to the rest of my life. I have been totally self-sufficient since I was seventeen years old. I was fearless and undaunted most of my life. There is no doubt in my mind that I was receiving instruction on humility and the sin of Pride. But here I was. Because of the way I felt I did not have any motivation to do anything which was not making my father too happy. To this day I do not think anyone in my family realized how sick I was. Time passed and it was finally time for me to have my surgery.

I was scheduled to have my surgery on the upcoming Monday. The Friday morning before, I was standing in the kitchen pouring a cup of coffee and as I looked to my left I saw my father standing on a ladder on the front porch. Suddenly the ladder tipped and he fell. He hit his hip on the edge of the concrete porch and shattered his hip. He had to have his hip replaced and would be in the hospital for some time. This created a situation for my mother who was not really capable of caring for herself. My father would be in the hospital and so would I. Fortunately, we were able to make arrangements for someone to stay with her but this meant I would be staying at my sister's after the surgery. My brother-in-law was not too happy. We get along great but I think he looked at it as an intrusion. We have never discussed it.

Monday came and into surgery I went. I knew this surgery was either going to save me or kill me. I was dreading having another abdominal surgery as they were far and above the most painful for me. The surgery was another long one. Twelve hours under the knife. The surgeon later told me she had found ten different fistulas inside me and so much infection in my abdomen she could not believe I was still alive. She told me she had basically gutted me like a fish. I then spent two weeks in ICU. As I knew it would be, the pain was horrific. My family and friends came to see me though which always helped. Finally it was time to go home to my sisters. I knew there would be tension and was really not able to do much so I just stayed in my room most of the time. The VA had arranged for in home nursing care and two nurses came to visit three times a week. They were amazed by the fact that I was in such good humor. I knew this was going to be another long healing process. About a month passed. My brother-in-law and sister had been talking to someone who had apparently told them I should be healed up by now and my brother-in-law was wondering when I was going to be leaving. He wondered what the problem was. Then I made a mistake, I borrowed a cigarette from a neighbor and he found out about it. Then I made the mistake of lying to him about the whole thing. He was furious and pulled out his bible and started reading to me about how much God hated liars and so on. I realized this was not so much about what I had done as it was about getting me out of his house.

I had another brother who lived about an hour south in Montgomery, Alabama. They called him and made arrangements for him to come pick me up and me to stay there. I was beginning to feel like a football being handed off from family member to family member. I do not mean to sound ungrateful as they all helped me at a time I would have had no other options, but I did not need their anger. I was doing everything I could just to maintain my sanity and fight to stay alive. My brother came to get me and I spent the next seven months at his house. He is pretty mellow but it was still an intrusion. The good news was, for the first time in several years, I was starting to feel better. This surgeon had done a great job and I really was optimistic about the future for the first time in a long time. I thanked God for this blessing and asked him to bless that surgeon too! I now had a permanent Colostomy and was now getting better and better with the passing of every week that went by. Again my hat goes off to the VA! I was flat broke and had no way to get any money. My brother was feeding me and letting me live in his house. He had enough problems of his own at the time so I kept as low a profile as I could. He worked second shift and slept during the day which created yet another conflict concerning noise. I had to be extremely quiet all day. I did a lot of praying and thinking during these months. Fortunately, my brother has an unbelievable library and I read one hundred twenty books while I was there. The funny thing was I had not picked up a book in years. I also was reading a Bible my sister had bought for me.

My wife and I had made an agreement when we separated that the following year we would sell the house and split any equity we had in it. It was now three years later and they were still living there. I had not pushed the fact that she had not followed our agreement because I knew she was struggling as I was not paying support since I had no income. I also wanted to make sure my children had a place to live. She was working but I had no idea what her income was. She had finally put the house up for sale but was not having much luck selling it. The market was still soft. The equity we had was a fair amount and I was counting on that money to return home and start over after my health got better. One day I got a letter from a court in Indiana. I opened the envelope to find papers stating that my wife had not made a payment on our house in nine months and the bank was repossessing our house. How could this be I wondered. She had not told me anything about not making payments. I had been talking with my kids on the phone and they had not mentioned anything to indicate that anything like this was happening either. I wondered just how many things can go wrong in a man's life. I was in a panic again. I needed that money to get a new start. I was picturing all sorts of things in my mind like being homeless or living a in a veteran's shelter the rest of my life or whatever. And none of the whatevers was good. Now as I have said over and over, God always takes care of me in a crisis. I guess maybe my faith was not as strong as I thought it was at this point or I would have realized that.

A couple of days later, my wife called me and much to my surprise, the house had sold. Talk about the old saying "In the nick of time". She needed a power of attorney from me to sell the house and said it was on its way. I signed and returned the document and waited to hear from her that the house had closed and to see how much money we would be splitting. I was so excited I remember. I would finally be able to return home and see my kids again. Then I got another surprise. As I was sitting there at my brother's one day, there was knock on the door and when I opened it, there was my son! I guess my family had made arrangements for him to come down for spring vacation. I was so happy I cried and cried. I was also shocked. I had not seen him in over two years and he had grown over a foot to a now towering six feet tall. To put that in perspective, I am five foot six and he was shorter than me by several inches when I left. The week passed quickly and he was gone again but it reminded me what I was living for again. I also knew that I would be able to leave and see them both again soon.

I waited and waited with no word from my wife about the sale of the house. She had told me that the house was closing on a certain date. That date had come and gone almost another week or two had passed. I awoke one Friday morning to a phone call from my banker in Indiana. I had maintained my account there since I knew I would eventually be returning home. My banker and I were good friends as I had known her since she was just a teller there and now she was the branch manager. She knew about my circumstances and the fact that I was living in Alabama. My wife had also opened an account for herself at the same bank after our separation. My banker said that she had three checks from a title company in her hand that had been deposited into my wife's accounts and they had my signature on them. She knew I had been living in Alabama and wondered if I had signed them. I told her no I did not know what she was talking about. She then said, "Then we have a problem". I am not going to go into the rest of the story but needless to say I got my half of the equity and now had the money I needed to go home.

I still had advanced stage COPD but I was no longer feeling sick all the time. My health was getting better and better every day. I started to exercise and was walking almost a mile every few days. I pushed myself hard to get back to health. This was not easy as humidity and COPD do not go together and I was in Alabama, one of the most humid states in the country. I was starting to experience some problems swallowing and so I went to the VA Hospital in Montgomery to the walk in clinic. I had been there several times since I had moved into my brother's house. They did an X-Ray of my neck. There was a small tumor in my neck which was protruding into my neck and creating the swallowing problems. I was optimistic because they told me it was very small and after a biopsy said that it was thyroid cells that had traveled down a blood vessel and located in my throat to form the tumor. They said they wanted to do some specialized Chemotherapy to try and shrink the tumor so they could remove it. They also said it had encapsulated itself in tissue and if all went well, it should be fairly easily removed with a somewhat minor surgery without any fear of it spreading. Well finally it seemed things were going my way a little for once. I would venture to say some of you are thinking, "How does having Cancer AGAIN in any way seem promising to this guy?"

When confronted with all this, I told the doctor that I had planned on heading home very shortly. He said he did not feel that would be a problem and they would transfer everything to my VA at home and make arrangements. Suddenly my life had changed dramatically. I had hope again for the first time in a long time. Even though I was confronted with Chemotherapy and yet another surgery, it seemed like a cake walk compared to what I had been through. There is an old saying, "Don't sweat the small sh..". I did not have a vehicle so I went shopping on line for a car. I finally found what I wanted and went to check it out. It was perfect and I even got it for great price. I was going home! Seeing my children again! I think I can honestly say it was one of the happiest moments I have ever experienced to this day.

CHAPTER XI

Going Home

The day finally came for me to go home. I was so excited to be seeing my kids again. It is about an eleven hour drive from Birmingham to home. I drove straight through except to stop for gas and food. I hit town and drove all the way around town straight to my daughter's house. I was in pretty bad shape when I got there because I had not done any breathing treatments all day and had smoked a pack of cigarettes on the way. I was so happy to see my daughter I began to cry. I was hardly able to breathe so I had her grab the Nebulizer from my car and we headed inside. She said we should go up to her room to do it. I was not thinking about the affect the stairs would have on me and was just about to the point of passing out by the time we got to the top. We got it plugged in and I began to draw the medicine in. Slowly but surely I began to feel my bronchial tubes begin to dilate. What a reunion I thought to myself. The first time I see my daughter in over two years and it has to be like this. I finally came around and I hugged her some more. I never wanted to let go. Unfortunately my worries of Cancer were quickly being replaced with anxiety about suffocation. I have often wondered how much of my subconscious is occupied by the suffocation issue.

I had made arrangements to stay with some friends of mine but that did not work out because they were now also having marital problems. I found a cheap hotel with weekly rates and ended up staying there a month. The hotel was a rat hole filled with welfare recipients living in poverty with no hope of changing their lives. Many were single mothers with children staying in what was basically an old motel room. Drugs and alcohol usage was rampant. I felt sorry for them and prayed for them. The cost of staying there a month was money I had not planned on spending. Even though I had the money from the house, I had no idea how long it would have to last and was trying to save every dime. The next day I went to the VA and had my records transferred from Birmingham and was assigned a new doctor. My new doctor was already overloaded and could not believe they would assign someone like me to her. I think the largest problem the VA has is its inability to keep doctors. She told me she had been reviewing my medical history and could not believe I was still alive. This was starting to be becoming a recurring theme with me and doctors and nurses. But I always replied with the same response, "The Big Guy upstairs has something he wants me to do".

She immediately scheduled me for blood work and some other tests so she could evaluate me. As I was leaving that day I saw many people that I knew. Everyone seemed shocked yet very happy to see me. I had left so suddenly that it seems many people had thought I had passed. They were also shocked at my marked improvement. Everyone kept telling me how great I looked. Almost every department at my VA Hospital has a nickname for me. Things like "The Miracle Man", "The Defiant One", "The Energizer Bunny" and my favorite, "The Cancer Killer". People, doctors and just about everyone thought it was some kind of miracle I was still alive. They would always make comments about my demeanor and my ability to maintain my sense of humor through all this. Soon a great many people began to tell me I should write a book. I would always laugh and tell them I was certainly no writer. I stopped by some of my old neighbors on the way home to say hello and see how they were. They were on the porch and when I got out of the car their mouths went open and they came up to me crying and hugging me. They also thought I had passed and had even spent time looking through obituaries at the library.

I must have heard just about every saying there is now. Things like you have used up twelve of your nine lives or so much for three strikes and you're out and so on. The more people went on, the more apparent my continued survival was a testament to God's love for me. About a month later I was able to find an apartment and began moving in. My furniture was in storage and I had some friends who did all the moving for me. I paid my rent for a year as I had no idea how long the money I had would last and I wanted to make sure I had a place to live for a while without worrying about paying the rent. I was just so thrilled to be home and seeing my kids again. I was soon contacted about my upcoming throat surgery and the Chemotherapy. I was dreading the thought of doing Chemotherapy again. I was pleasantly surprised to find out it would be for only a short period of time and was nothing like my previous experience. We waited for the Chemotherapy to work on the tumor. It was very successful and a short time later I was having the surgery on my throat. It was like a walk in the park compared to what I had experienced in the past. It seemed things were looking up a little for the first time in a long time. My stay in the hospital was short one this time. I was only there a few days. I was starting to have hope about the future and was thanking God for his continued love and caring for me. I am amazed at the resilience of the human body and spirit to survive what seems to be insurmountable odds. As I said before, "God made us Strong!"

This is a little out of sequence but it just goes to prove the statement I just made. A couple of days ago during the writing of this book I began to experience some lower back and abdominal pain. I knew it was not related to anything that has happened so far and to make a long story short, I had Pancreatitis and had to have my Gaul Bladder removed. It was the seventh, yes seventh body part they have now thrown in the trash can. As I lay waiting for the Anesthesiologist to come start the "Juice" as I now called it, a nurse was holding my hand and saying, "Don't worry it will be alright". The surgeon was chuckling as the nurse made her comment. This was the surgeon who had put my intestines back in previously. She said, "Honey this is going to be like having his tonsils removed for this guy". She looked down at me and winked. We arrived at the operating room and the anesthesiologist and I had a brief conversation. A moment later everything went dark. The surgery went perfectly and I soon found myself home again.

Summer passed and fall was upon us. I love fall in Indiana because it is so colorful. I missed the four distinct seasons we have in Indiana while I was down south. By this point the money was quickly running out and I knew I had to find a job of some kind. The problem was my COPD was going to make that very difficult not to mention no one wants to hire someone who had the medical problems I had. As I keep saying, every time things become a crisis, God steps in and takes care of me. I was driving across a parking lot at the store one day when I saw an old friend of mine who owned a bowling alley that I had worked at part time many years ago. I stopped to say hello. After a few pleasantries he noticed the scar on my neck and asked what had happened. I explained about the Cancer and all. He asked me where I was working and I told him I had just got back to town shortly before that and was not working due to the limitations of my COPD. Well, guess what, he had a job for me. Another coincidence I guess.

I would not get rich but with the assistance I was getting from SNAP I was able to at least survive. A short time later my breathing started becoming more and more difficult. I was still smoking but I did not think that was it. I knew what COPD attacks were by this point. I also felt like my skin was crawling and my heart was constantly palpitating any time I exerted myself. I knew it was something different this time. I found my answer quite by accident one morning as I was taking my thyroid medication. As I looked at the bottle I discovered they had changed the amount of medication that was in each tablet and I was supposed to be cutting them in half. So here I had been double dosing my Thyroid medication for over two months now. I immediately called the doctor. The problem was, this had also made me irritable and had created a great deal of friction between my boss and me at work. I was let go shortly thereafter. I was again in a panic about money. I was also a mess from the whole medication overdose problem. Well, it was nice while it lasted.

After I got my medication regulated I was wondering what I was going to do. I did manage to get two more little jobs but was let go from both because of my breathing difficulties. I was in full panic mode again. I found myself having to get help with my rent from the Township Trustees office and was selling just about everything I had that was not tied down. I was getting further and further behind on the rent and knew it was just a matter of time before I got an eviction notice. It suddenly occurred to me. I had found out about a VA pension a short time before I had left for Alabama. I had applied but had never followed up on it after I left. I do not like taking money from the government. There is always a catch you know. But these were Veteran's Benefits that I had earned through my time in the service. The following Monday I went to the VA office down at the court house and talked to a gentleman about it. He was more than happy to help me out and he was able to do all the paperwork right through his VA computer which would speed things up he said. Again, I had a little hope. It was not a lot of money, but it in combination with other programs and assistance I was eligible for since I was now considered totally disabled, I would be able to pay my bills and not starve to death. I also found out about a state program called SSI.

In the end I was approved for both but was only able to collect the VA Pension. I was so happy to find out I was approved in only two weeks! I was amazed at the speed at which they were back to me. They said since I was Vietnam Era veteran, was 70% disabled and had no hope to obtain gainful employment, I was approved. It did take some time to get caught up but at least I did not now have to worry being homeless. There is no way I can express the anxiety I had been experiencing before that. Financial issues in combination with the anxiety about breathing had made me a mess. My doctor decided I needed a little help and put me on an anti-anxiety drug. I was still making trips to the VA ER for COPD attacks. Of course I was still smoking and was not willing to admit that this was really the cause of my breathing problems. Last year, the day before my birthday, I was sitting home playing on my laptop when I coughed.

Some mucus came up but was blocking my airways. I kept coughing very hard in an effort to remove the obstruction. My muscles were becoming fatigued and then soon, I was no longer able to cough. My muscles began to cramp creating great pain on top of the suffocating and I could not breathe.

I threw down the computer and headed to the kitchen where my Nebulizer is. I got about half way to the kitchen and I could feel my muscles giving out. I went to my knees. Then Hypoxia began to set in and my temples began to burn. Hypoxia is when the body becomes deprived of oxygen. This of course includes the brain. I felt myself fading as if I was going to pass out. I managed to crawl to the kitchen and was reaching up onto the counter for the parts to my Nebulizer when my bladder cut loose. My bladder emptied and I was now lying on the floor in a puddle of urine. I am not really sure how I managed to do it, but somehow I got the Nebulizer parts put together and the medicine loaded and was able to take some breathes. I now keep my Nebulizer assembled and full of medicine at all times as it may make the difference between life and death as I was finding out. One, then two, then three breathes until I was finally able to think again. I continued to take as deep of breathes as I could and then I grabbed my Steroid inhaler and hit it too. I was able to recover enough to get to my car and head for the VA Emergency Room. I am fortunate in that I can make it to the VA Emergency Room in about four or five minutes if I drive fast.

Upon arrival it the ER they did all the usual things and I was soon feeling much better. They always take good care of me there. After discussing what had happened with the doctor, he told me it sounded like I did not have but a minute or two and I probably would have been dead. As you can see, I am my own worst enemy. These kinds of experiences have become a part of my life and I have just learned to accept them. I was again finding myself thanking God for my continued existence. I was now starting to find myself embarrassed in front of God. He kept saving me and I kept smoking and doing everything wrong. I remembered a story in the bible about a man whose plight was similar. He was ashamed because God kept saving him and he kept screwing up. That was exactly how I was feeling at that moment. I continually find myself wondering what God is saving me for. I have told him I am willing to do anything he needs me to do. After all, how many times has he saved me now? Too many to count!

I am not sure how many times events occur during the writing of a book that are actually relevant to the topic of the book but something else has happened. It does not really have to do with Cancer, but to my everlasting struggle to persevere, with God's help of course. I recently found I had a condition known as Bell's Palsy on the left side of my face. They gave me some antibiotics and steroids. It lasted about three weeks and went away. Two months later it came back on the other side of my face. I am fortunate that with treatment it went away but I cannot help wondering why I cannot seem to learn the lesson that it is becoming obvious that God is trying to teach me. In case you did not know it, I am going for the Guinness World Book of Records for having had the most diseases and body parts a man can have removed and still live!

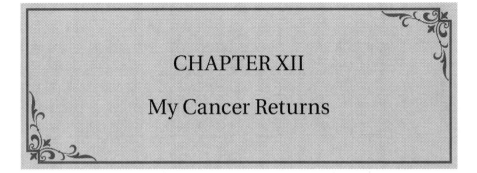

CHAPTER XII

My Cancer Returns

I cannot help but wonder if some of you are starting to think my story is a fiction. How can this guy still be alive you are probably asking yourself. Cancer kills everyone you know. Overall, this year has not been a bad one so far. I always include a "Caveat" when making any statements that imply anything about the future. This year I have had to make fewer trips to the ER for COPD attacks. Recently I was scheduled for a regular appointment with my regular doctor. As usual, there was the blood work that is always done prior. Since I do not have a Thyroid Gland and take the "Synthroid" mentioned earlier, and considering my history with Thyroid Cancer, the levels of Thyroid in my system are monitored every time they draw blood. When I went to the appointment, my doctor was concerned. The tests had come back showing elevated thyroid levels in my system. I was fairly sure I knew what this meant recalling the earlier ultrasound I had showing the lymph node in my neck on the right side a few years ago. I was referred to an Endocrinologist for further consultation and testing. I told him about the lymph node they had found years before. He decided it was time to do another ultrasound of my neck.

A few weeks later I reported for the test. The technicians are not allowed to say anything, but I knew she had found something by the number of pictures she was taking. I short time later I met with the Endocrinologist again to discuss the results. It now appeared that there were four lymph nodes containing Cancer. I think my anticipation of this happening at some point in the future lessened the impact of this news. I have also come to feel that God had not helped me through all this just to let me get sick and die now. I guess I am learning what faith really is. I took the news fairly well although I also knew what it meant. More testing and surgery and I knew both would involve more pain. I was still confused as to why God was keeping me alive and holding me giving me strength. But I love him and thank him for his love and protection. I know I am very excited by the prospect of doing something for him. I hear people speak of a plan that God has for all of us. At this time in my life I believe I am seeing that come to fruition right before my very eyes. As human beings we just cannot fathom what he may see as our own destinies in life unfold, but I am very much looking forward to whatever my destiny is. I love and thank God for my very existence every day. I talk to him constantly as I spend a great deal of time by myself which makes it easy to do.

I was told I would again need to go to the Roudebush Medical Center in Indianapolis. A few weeks later I reported for the consult. The doctors had reviewed the ultrasound and had a many questions. Sometimes I get frustrated because most of the answers to their questions are in their computer if they would just take the time to read it. Again, these two doctors seemed to be amazed at my continued survival. I responded with the usual. I have found that doctors and nurses are very quiet when it comes to the powers of healing associated with faith in God. Most of them are people of science and I believe for a lot of them, it is beyond their scope of understanding. After the consult they told me I would have to return the following week for a biopsy. Most biopsies are not fun and involve a certain amount of pain. This particular kind of biopsy was no exception.

They would be doing what is known as a "Fine Needle Aspiration" or FNA as they like to call it. I was already familiar with the procedure as I had it done on the other side of my neck previously and it was also the procedure they had used to check my goiters earlier. This procedure involved taking a needle and plunging it repeatedly into the lymph node to collect the cells inside the needle. And I do mean repeatedly. They are actually scraping the cells into the inside of the needle by the repeated plunging action. Not fun I must say. Even though they do a local anesthetic, it still hurts. I cannot remember why, but they cannot just suck the cells into the syringe for some reason. They must be scraped into the needle by the repeated plunging action. After I finished the FNA, I went home and played the waiting game again.

It did not take much time for me to get the bad news. Each of the four lymph nodes contained Cancerous Thyroid cells. They would have to perform another surgery similar to the one they had done on the other side of my neck. They had done the lab work and it was definitely Cancer. Particulate Thyroid Cancer cells had migrated into four lymph nodes and had multiplied considerably. This time they would take no chances and would be performing what they called a "Right Modified Radical Neck Dissection". Now that certainly got my attention. The word dissection made me think about the ninth grade and that poor frog we "Dissected" in Biology class. Then there was the phrase "Modified Radical". I was not bad enough that it was "Radical", it was SO radical, they had to "Modify" it! The extent of the removal of the lymph nodes would be greater than in my first neck dissection and this one would also involve making a second incision paralleling the collar bone.

I was again given some warnings about nerve damage. I was told there is a major nerve bundle running through the area where they would be performing the surgery. He warned that there may be some partial paralysis in the right arm as a result of the surgery. I have said it before; it just gets better and better! I joke because at this point, I have no doubt my faith in God will pull me through. As I describe events that pass, have you noticed the change in my comfort levels as my faith in God has increased? At the same time, I do not want to appear complacent and assuming. Feeling that I do not have to worry and assume he will take care of me no matter what. Never take the Lord for granite. You must still pray and do right by the Lord. I am not really sure how well I am doing as far as that last part is concerned, but I sure am trying hard. Maybe that is what he needs to see to keep his faith in me and knows that I will overcome my downfalls eventually.

I reported back to Indy the following week for my surgery. It would only last five hours. This would be a quickie for me so to say. The main incision would start just below the end of the other scar on my neck and follow around and up the other side of my neck to behind the right ear. There would also be and four inch long incision paralleling my collar bone. I would no longer have a cockeyed grin but a full smile under my smile! Now it looks like a guy smiling with a cigarette hanging out of his mouth. How ironic. Maybe I will have a little smoke tattooed at the end of the scar that looks like the cigarette. I must say though, it does look like someone slit my throat from ear to ear. I remember shortly after my first neck surgery I was standing in line at the store and there was a little boy about four or so in line in front of me with his mother. He was looking at me very intensely then he tugged on his mom's pants and she bent over and he tried to whisper in her ear. I heard him say, "Mommy, that man got robbed". She asked him what made him think that and he replied that they had slit my throat doing it. I laughed and told him that I had cancer and the doctors had made the scars he saw. He asked me if I was ok now and I told him yes. He seemed somehow relieved to hear that. I love children. They bring so much joy and you just never what is coming out of their mouth next! Again the pain and discomfort was similar to the of my first neck dissection. That was to include the constant feeling of being choked as the scar tissue started to form inside. Also, with all the discussion about Opioid addiction these days, they are a little reluctant to give them in similar doses as my first neck surgery and thus the pain was a little more severe. Also do you remember my "Morphine Clicker" I had in previous surgeries? That was not to be either. Again I had thirty or so staples in my neck.

I only had to spend four days in the hospital recovering this time. I was glad to get home when it was over. There's no place like home as Dorothy said in the Wizard of Oz. The comfort of one's own bed is nothing to be compared to. I also knew there would be more follow up appointments soon to follow. I believe I ended up making trips to Indianapolis five out of six weeks during this period. My next trip was the usual post-surgery follow up to observe my progress. The doctor was amazed at how fast I was healing. He told me with all that I had been through, he was somewhat concerned about post-surgery pneumonia due to lack of a strong immune system. I have had so many comments made at this point referring to my strengths, they sort of go in one ear and out the other. I remember he made the comment, "I don't know what you are eating, but we need to start feeding it to all the Oncology patients." Remember, we must keep our sense of humor. I am sure many of you out there are familiar with a magazine called "The Readers Digest". When I was very young, I used to sit at my grandmother's house and read it. There was one regular section that appeared every month called "Laughter is the Best Medicine". I have never forgotten that.

My final appointment involved some more very extensive tests. One was the test I mentioned in an earlier chapter involving the radio-active Isotope 123. The other was the full body P.E.T. Scan I also mentioned before. I was now going to have those two tests again. Considering my continued smoking, I was a little fearful of what the PET scan might show. From previous experience, I knew you could have a tumor in your lung and never even know it. I had been seven years without the Lung Cancer returning. That is a miracle in itself. I had to wait three days for the test results. I prayed and prayed to God to let the tests show I was still Cancer free. When the results came in, my prayers were answered. There was no sign of Cancer anywhere in my body. After all that I have been through and all the Cancer that has been in my body, how can you possibly believe at this point that there has not been some kind of Divine Intervention in my life. Cancer Free! You cannot imagine what those words mean to someone who has been afflicted with this horrible disease. When I got the news I cried and thanked the Lord. I am still so confused though. How can this be that a sinner like me has been picked by God to survive. I am beginning to think he does it just to show me how forgiving he can be even in the case of extreme sinners like me. Only he knows why, but I will stay ever vigilant in my fight and continue my faith knowing that he has a reason for keeping me alive and when he calls, I will be gladly waiting to help.

Some time has passed again and I seem to be doing pretty well. I am still in constant conflict over my smoking. I have also recently discovered I have yet another condition called "Cough Syncope". When I cough extremely hard, occasionally there is a response caused by what is known as the Vagus nerve. It causes me to almost pass out and my left side goes into convulsions almost like an epileptic seizure. It matters not, I will continue on and live life to the very fullest I can.

CHAPTER XIII

A Chapter for Smokers

I have continued to smoke through this whole ordeal. I am sure that you who do not smoke are wondering what kind of idiot I am. Stupid does as stupid is. I have tried just about every method and trick there is to try and stop. I have told myself only this many a day and all those other little tricks we smokers try. Problem is, as soon as you light that FIRST cigarette up, you are done. Those of you who do smoke and tell yourself all those things you tell yourself to justify your continued use of tobacco, know exactly what I mean. I was using my illness as an excuse to continue smoking. I would tell people, "With all I have been through and all the stress, it has not been a good time to try and quit". As you can see, all I was doing was compounding my problems over and over. We tolerate all of the destructiveness to ourselves and our belongings. It is pain we inflict on our loved ones who watch us slowly destroy ourselves. I am the poster boy for destroying one's own health. It is the burnt clothes, furniture and car seats. Some people even have fallen asleep and caught themselves or homes on fire. And that is not to mention the smell. Everything we own smells like that damn smoke. I have made so many trips to the ER for "Exasperated COPD attacks" I cannot even count the number. This usually involves shots of steroids and a prescription, which for some is just more money out of their pockets.

As I have said before in this book, it is amazing what we can do with our minds. Unfortunately, that can sometimes work against us in a negative way as you can see in this case. I continued to tell myself I can will my way through all this the way as I have in the past. The problem is, when I am doing this, God is not with me giving me his help. He will not help me destroy my own body, his temple. It is the gift of life that I am not respecting. This week, I found myself in dire straits. I was smoking way too much and not getting the sleep I needed. I developed a sinus infection. I just thought it was the usual stuffy nose I get sometimes. Saturday afternoon I suddenly found myself hardly able to breathe. I knew I needed to get to the ER. I received the usual treatment and was on my way. Little did I know that you can only cheat for so long before God will teach you a lesson. The following afternoon I was struck again with another COPD attack. I could not breathe. I ran for my Nebulizer and spent the next three hours on it fighting for every breath. I knew something was different this time. I never had these attacks two days in a row. It was so bad I actually considered calling an ambulance. That was something I had never done before. I was panicking and afraid to put the Nebulizer down. After three hours of sucking on that nebulizer, I was finally able to get my Steroid inhaler and caught my breathe enough to get to the VA. By the time I got there, I was suffocating. It was so bad this time that they were considering putting me on a respirator. Being hooked up to a respirator is not something you want to go through. Fortunately, I was able to recover just enough that they decided not to do it. Thank God again! But I did realize from their reactions, this time was different than any previous visits.

It seems that this was not only a problem with my COPD but the sinus infection had migrated down the back of my throat into my lungs and was compounding my breathing problems. Every time my lungs fill up with the stuff, it made it hard to catch my breath. They decided to admit me to the hospital. I have now been in ICU for eight days with no end in sight. I sit on the edge of my bed most of the time panting like a dog on a hot summer day trying to get enough oxygen to maintain. They are also confused as to why I am not bouncing back as I usually do. They are pumping me full of steroids and are now on a second type of antibiotic. They seem to be trying this and that but I am not turning around. I am actually writing this as I lay in bed at the hospital. I stand to use the toilet which is only five feet away and by the time I get there I am almost passing out. They seem to be testing everything. I am coughing up the greenest stuff you ever saw but the tests are coming back negative for a bacterial infection. So that leaves fungal and viral infections. I am scared this time. I will keep you posted, or maybe not according to how this plays out. I guess something could happen here that keeps me from finishing this book.

The thing about smoking addiction is that it actually consists of two parts. The first is the obvious physical addiction to Nicotine that almost everyone knows about. The addiction that leads to all of the health issues associated with smoking. The second is the mental addiction. I like to call this the "Cultural Addiction". This is the one you do not hear about on all those commercials for products sold to help people stop smoking. In my case, this is the dominant of the two. Smoking is a culture. It is as much a part of our lives as breathing and eating. We associate and support each other's bad habit. It almost reinforces the fact that in our minds, this is alright to do. People who do not smoke just do not understand this part of the equation. Unfortunately the effects of smoking are not immediate and slowly take us over at a point that it is extremely hard to stop this habit because we have smoked for so long. As I said, it is as much a part of us as eating or breathing. The problem is you may not be able to do the later for very long if you smoke long enough. I have heard from others all the excuses they use to justify their smoking. It will not happen to me I am very healthy and in good shape. No one in my family has ever had Cancer or the old it is genetics thing. But eventually, you WILL feel the negative effects of smoking. That includes everything from extreme shortness of breath to full blown Lung Cancer or Heart Disease. I am not your daddy, but do yourself a favor, QUIT!

Just the expense alone is becoming rather exorbitant. And that cost is only going to rise. The government is trying to tax you out of your habit now and no one feels sorry for you having to pay more taxes for your cigarettes because it is what is known as a "Sin Tax". And I certainly hope you are not looking for sympathy from the non-smoking or anti-smoking crowds. They already hate you because you stink and invade their air space. I see people at the gas station or smoke shop buying cigarettes and so many look like the people that can afford them the least. In Indiana, if you smoke one pack of cigarettes a day, it is costing you anywhere from one hundred eighty to two hundred twenty five dollars a month to smoke according to brand. In many states like New York the cost is even greater as the state taxes are much more. And think of the cost if you smoke two or even three packs a day. That is one hell of a lot of money to pay to kill yourself! Damn man, that is a car or house payment! And another thing, no matter how much it costs, a smoker will ALWAYS find a way to support his habit. I remember there was a period of time when I was pretty broke and I would get in my car and drive around bumming cigarettes from anyone I saw smoking. I could collect a pack in a half hour to an hour. We all have our stresses in life and smoking is just one of the many stress relieving habits that people have. It just seems that all those habits seem to kill us. I know my son and daughter have certainly suffered greatly. Every time I light up my daughter cries and my son scowls. It seems we love our cigarettes more than we love ourselves and our loved ones. The suffering that my children have been through and continue to go through because of my smoking is horrible. If nothing else, do it for them!

So, having said this, I have a decision to make. RIGHT NOW as I lay in this hospital bed. I have started the patch, which I have never tried before, and not being able to smoke in the hospital will give me a good start. As usual, God is letting me take myself to the brink before I learn the lesson and he reaches into the bowels of death and pulls me free. Notice I said take MYSELF to the brink, not GOD taking me to the brink. I do and will always associate these horrible things we do to Satan and temptation. The difference is whether WE decide to resist or participate in the temptation. I am weak in this regard and I know it. God has given me so many great abilities that I threw away to temptation. What a waste. I have just been told

I am moving to the regular ward shortly. Guess I am going to be here a while.

I am going to continue to add to this chapter as I continue the writing of this book. It will be a real time example where you see the real time results. I will pray and I have faith God will help me through this if I am sincere in my efforts. I think I have finally said to myself, "Enough is enough!" I am sick of the coughing and pain. The suffocating and anxiety associated with suffocation. My sixteen year old is cautious and says, "We will see dad, you are not able to smoke here. We will see after you get home". Smart kid. One thing I do know. I will never have to worry about my kids smoking after the nightmare they have lived through their father. I think I have finally come to the point where the accumulation of everything has finally brought me where I CAN do this. If I want to go on living, I must quit this horrible trek I have been on. I was basically told the other day that if I do not quit, in six months I will be Oxygen dependent and subject to the all the limitations that go with it. In five years or so, enough of my Alveoli will be damaged that my lungs will no longer be able to process enough Oxygen to keep my body alive. Well, that statement hit home pretty hard! Alveoli are the little sacks in your lungs that process the air that we breathe. They extract the oxygen from the air and put it into the blood system.

I guess this is going to be my "Significant Emotional Event", as psychologists call it that may actually change my life. At this moment I am exhausted from panting like a dog for six straight days and constantly wondering if my heart may give out or I will just suffocate. Suffocation is something that has to be experienced to understand. There is extreme panic that hits your mind and body. There is pain and weakness that quickly sets in when the body is deprived of all oxygen. And I live my life surrounded with such attacks and the anxiety of wondering when the next time will come. Believe me folks it is NO WAY TO LIVE!

Earlier I mentioned a time before that I said I had made a promise to God and then did not keep it. I truly believe that breaking that promise may be partially responsible for me being here now. The other day as I sat there on my Nebulizer, and even though I had vowed never to make a promise to God again due to my weakness, I again made a promise to God that if he would just get me through this, I would quit smoking. At that time I made the earlier promise, I was not nearly the spiritual person I am now. There is no doubt in my mind that the promise I just made will be the single greatest motivator to my quitting. I will live in fear of what will happen if I start again. I am much stronger in my faith now and understand that if I am sincere in my desire to quit, God will help me. I know there are those of you who are saying that this is just a ploy I am using to get myself to quit. I said I do not believe in coincidence, I think everything happens for a reason. I am sure you have heard the saying that sometimes God works in strange ways and I am sure that saying applies in total to all the idiots like me who keep smoking even after being through what I have. I cannot help but wonder that God realizes my weakness in regards to my smoking and put me here for twelve days with no ability to smoke just to give me the head start I needed to be able to succeed. WE SHALL SEE!

I hope that some of you will use my misery and suffering, and that of my family to reflect on your own lives and families and what smoking has done, is doing and will do to you and them. I never thought I would be an advocate for the anti-smoking crowd. I have smoked for forty seven years now and am a very staunch believer in individual freedom and personal rights. Yet it breaks my heart to see all of you out there that are suffering because you could not quit something that is slowly killing you. Well, I am now four days out of ICU. Something seems to be changing today. My immune system (what is left of it) must be starting to have an effect. I am breathing a little better today and the mucus is almost clear. I am sure it does not hurt that I have now been without a cigarette for twelve days. They have removed my oxygen and tomorrow they say if I can do the six minute walk and keep my oxygen levels above ninety percent, I can go home. I am so excited. It is amazing what twelve days without smoke can do for your lungs. The inflammation seems to be almost subsided and the mucus levels are minimal. I am still coughing stuff up but they tell me that is natural for someone who stops smoking. I also feel like I have a decent amount of air moving through my lungs. I also used to cough from morning until night and I am hardly coughing at all. I cannot help but wonder what it will be like in a couple of months, a year and so on. No cigarettes and getting some exercise will make me a new man I bet! I should get on my knees and thank God for pulling me from the depths again. And I WILL keep that promise.

I am going to have a little plaque made for above my stove that says "THE PROMISE" so that every morning when I pour that cup of coffee, I will be reminded. Not that I could forget. I think fear of what will happen if I break my promise and the desire to get well will keep me in line. I must also mention that yet again I am saved. Are you beginning to understand my feelings about God? Do you really think that I am that strong or the medicine saved me? I love the doctors, but they were running all those tests and coming up empty handed remember. And even though they were trying the antibiotics, remember they told me all the tests indicated that there was no bacterial infection. I guess for some of you, it is just another coincidence or more of my luck I guess.

I have now been home for nine days. I have not smoked in twenty one days and I have been Nicotine free for a week. The difference is I was on the patch which still puts nicotine into your system. But not smoking any cigarettes for three weeks is a major accomplishment for me. The thing is I am experiencing no craving or desire to go buy a pack. I knew if I did not buy one within two days of coming home, I had this licked. I want to tell you a few of the great things I am experiencing at the twenty one day mark. The improvements in my breathing are extremely dramatic. Before I went into the hospital, I could not walk a hundred feet without stopping to catch my breath. Yesterday I walked over to coffee shop that is about a quarter of a mile from my house at two o'clock in the afternoon and it was 85 degrees and the humidity was sixty seven percent, and I did not stop a single time. My recovery time was less than three minutes. A month ago there was no way I would have even considered such a thing. Today,

I walked to the grocery that is about a half mile from my house, it was cooler today and overcast so I am sure that helped but again I did not stop once and I carried home two bags of groceries, one of which probably weighed about twenty five pounds. This morning I took a shower for the first time I can remember without dreading it and with very little effort. Yesterday I ran up the stairs and came back down before it occurred to me that I had done it without sitting down for five minutes with my heart pounding and breathing like that panting dog I always mention. Another thing happened today. I caught myself singing. Because of the effects the smoking has had on my vocal chords, I have not been able to sing for a long time. It may sound silly but it really made my day.

This morning I woke up and realized that something was very different. Something that I could not put my finger on had also occurred. Then it hit me. For the first time in seven years, I was not feeling that underlying sense of fear and anxiety about suffocation. I will say, when I came to this epiphany, I broke down and cried. This will actually be the greatest benefit to me out of them all. Yes even more than the better breathing. I actually sat here trying to come up with an analogy or description for this feeling, but I could not find anything that describes the feeling of being free of that mental burden. I thanked God the moment I realized what has happened. I really wish I could duplicate this feeling and give it to smokers. The feeling of all the things I have just described. If you could show smokers the contrast between then and now, everyone would be quitting. I have not even mentioned how much more energy I have and how great I feel. It is some kind of a high I have never heard of. I am enthusiastic about the future again. My children and everyone I know are thrilled for me. People tell me how great I look and some have even made jokes about my caffeine consumption because I am so exuberant and full of energy. This is not to mention that my apartment and car no longer smell like an ash tray. I just cannot help but wonder if this is happening in only three weeks, what will down the road three months, or even three years be like? I can only imagine at this point. I do know one thing, I will never pick up a cigarette again. I have also figured out that telling yourself I will only have one, is a recipe for your failure. Never again!

As I said, I am going to leave this chapter open until I am ready to publish so that I may continue to let you realize the benefits real time as they are happening. It had now been thirty days since I quit. It seems that with the passing of every week now, there seems to be some type of major improvements. I am now noticing my focus and concentration have improved. I am sure that is for two reasons. One I am now getting more Oxygen to the brain. Two, I am not experiencing the anxiety which was a constant distraction to clear thinking. My short term memory also seems to be improving. I seem to be able to quickly recall things better than I have for some time. Energy levels are continuing to increase. I am on the last twenty days of the antiviral treatment for my Hepatitis C treatment which is supposed to suppress energy levels to some extent. So I cannot help but wonder what my energy levels will be like after I complete the treatment and am no longer taking the medication. At that point I will be almost sixty days without a cigarette and I can only imagine what my energy levels will be like. And now for you people who like to eat. Everything, and I do mean everything, seems to taste delicious. Food seems to have so much more flavor and I am eating things I would never have dreamed of eating a month ago. It has been 40 days now with no cigarettes and I feel fabulous. This will be my last post before I finish and get ready for publication. Do yourself a favor and get rid of those cigarettes!

CHAPTER XIV

Parents of Children with Cancer

I was sitting and watching television last night when a commercial for one of the children's Cancer hospitals came on. It suddenly occurred to me that I had not included them in my book. If you knew me you would know this was a terrible omission on my part because I love children so much. They are our most precious resource and our future. There is nothing like the smile and laugh of a child to make one feel good. So I decided to do a little bit of a rewrite to finalize the book. You will see how much I care for these kids in the last paragraph of this book. I know the suffering I have endured during my battle with cancer and I am an adult so I cannot imagine what it must be like to be six or seven years old and have someone tell me I have Cancer. Here their life is just getting started and they are told it may end before they ever get to experience all the wonderful things life has to offer. I am sure it must seem extremely unfair to them. Some of them probably wonder what they did wrong to deserve this. Parents have so much to overcome with these children. I also know I cannot begin to understand how someone who is told that their child has been diagnosed with Cancer must feel. Having said that I can only try to say a few words to try and make both feel a little better and possibly help them in their battle. I can relate to the love we feel for our children and the horrible effect this disease has on family's lives. My daughter is now twenty years old. She was only six and my son was three when my battle started. She says even though she knows how important this book is to me she refuses to read the first fourteen chapters. She said she just does not want to go through all that suffering again. I saw the tears in her eyes and can only imagine the memories that must have passed through her head when I handed her a copy of the book on a thumb drive to read. Seeing her reaction all these years later makes me wonder how a parent who has a child with Cancer must feel. She was not really able to understand other than daddy has a terrible disease.

Most often the child does not understand and according to their age, is just plain scared to death. Parents DO understand all that goes with this disease. They are the ones who are fully informed by the doctors and have to make the difficult decisions concerning the future of their child. I am sure that does not make the emotions of dealing with it any easier either. I can tell you some of the decisions you will have to make will not be easy so prepare yourself to deal with it ahead of time. To most, their children are the most precious things in their lives. And to find out their child has a disease that may take their child from them must be something that cannot be put into words. To have to sit and watch your child suffer day in and day out sometimes for years. I do not think there are really words to describe it. The thought of our child suffering and possibly losing their life to this disease has got to be one of the most devastating things a person can experience in life. As I said before, the child may have very little understanding as to what Cancer is. This is where the parents and doctors must exercise great care and wisdom in how they present the subject to the child. Some of the older ones will have read or even possibly known someone who died of Cancer. They must be made to understand that no matter what they have read or who they have known it is totally irrelevant to their situation and that they understand that every case is different. As you have read you know how important it is to make sure your child is filled with determination and fight. Everyone must make sure they understand that there is always hope. A lot of that will come from how it is presented to them. Some are babies born with the disease and never know any different. Every situation is especially different when it comes to the children. They are not mentally developed yet and are so susceptible to how all this is presented to them and believe me they pay a lot of attention to what is going on around them. They are little sponges that soak up everything around them.

Obviously babies and toddlers will have no understanding of what is going on medically but I can guarantee you they can sense the emotional part. I cannot stress the importance of making sure that everyone around them maintains an uplifting attitude when they are around them. Sitting and crying in front of them is being selfish. I know that it may sound cold for me to say that, but you must think of how they feel and not how you feel. If you want to make sure your child has every chance to get through this they must have everything possible going for them. You have read how I feel about keeping that positive mental attitude through all this. You must help make them strong mentally. This has to be done in a way that is very delicate because I am sure there is a fine line between whether they perceive all this in a negative or positive way. You must learn what makes them really happy and when they are down use that to help them struggle through mentally. Will that always be possible? Of course not because they are a child with little understanding of what is really happening. Most of what they understand is what they see and what they sense emotionally from those around them. My heart goes out to these parents. I cannot think of anything more trying and emotionally devastating than having a child with Cancer. YOU are one of the keys to how they deal with this mentally and emotionally. I firmly believe that keeping them going and fighting is half the battle.

Try to create an environment that is as cheerful and comfortable as possible. I would think making their hospital room as much like home as possible would be part of this. According to what the hospital will allow, bring as much of home to their hospital room as possible. Bring them their special toys, maybe their "Blankie" or their favorite books and movies. Take them an MP3 player or device to play their favorite songs on. If possible buy or borrow a portable DVD player to play their favorite movies on. Bring everything that you can to make it seem more like home. This will help them emotionally and make them feel more comfortable. It will help reduce stress and they need all the help they can get. When you are with them make sure you are fully engaged in making that time be as happy and loving for them as possible. I know this will not be easy and I am sure that after a period of time this may become very hard to do. I am sure this is especially true if the child's prognosis is not favorable. You must think of this from the standpoint that this is the only time they may have left in their life and you want to make it as loving, wonderful and special as possible. I know how much I love my children and if it was me in this situation, I would do ANYTHING to make them happy. You MUST maintain this attitude when you are in their presence for their sake. You can always deal with your emotions when you get home.

Speaking of the emotion of all this, I would like to mention something I have been reading about that may cheer a few of you up and give you and them hope. Optimism can be very contagious! I have been reading about a very new treatment that seems to be very successful for some children with cancer. It has been especially successful for children with Leukemia. From what I have seen and read, Leukemia seems to be one of the most prevalent forms of Cancer in children. There is a new treatment called "CAR T". This is part of a rapidly emerging immunotherapy called ACT (Adoptive Cell Transfer). I am certainly not a doctor but there is a lot of information on the internet about it. I know if I were a parent of a child with Cancer I would be exhausting EVERY avenue I could to try and save my child. Without getting too technical, this treatment involves engineering your child's own immune cells to fight the disease. Not all forms have been approved by the FDA but sometimes there are ways around that. It HAS been approved for children with Acute Lymphoblastic Leukemia. I have also read about several other successes for treating other types of Leukemia. Usually when a new method of treatment is discovered there is a great deal of pressure applied to hurry the process of approval when it comes to saving children's lives. There is a great deal of research going on when it comes to children with Cancer. I would discuss some of these new treatments with your child's Oncologist. You must stay informed regarding new treatments.

To put it as delicately as possible, doctors are human beings too and they make mistakes. Remember this is your precious child's life. You should NEVER be afraid to get a second opinion if something does not seem quite right. Sometimes insurance companies may not have approved a new treatment yet or possibly your child's hospital may not have approved it. I do not know them all, but I am sure there are a great many barriers that can be there when it comes to new treatments. Sometimes there are ways around that such as volunteering for clinical trials or if need be, move your child to a hospital where they DO allow a certain treatment. I am in no way advocating that you do any of these things without doing it properly and only with your child's life saving interests in mind. ALWAYS consult Oncologists for the best way to proceed. Almost any type of new treatment involves a certain amount of or maybe even a lot of risk. ONLY your child's Oncologist can help you make informed decisions. I just know that if I had a five your old child with Cancer I would do anything to save them. Remember my statement a moment ago about having tough decisions to make? Well this is one of those kinds of decisions I was talking about.

Now I want to touch on a part of your child's treatment that some will agree with and some will not. For those of you who do not agree, I can only say that if you have read this whole book you know I feel without a doubt that there is a spiritual part to healing. Even though you or your child may not really comprehend this aspect of healing, I know someone who does and that is God. I believe God does sometimes work in strange ways as the saying goes. I do know I would not be here writing this if it were not for him. Do you not want your child to have EVERY chance to live and be healthy? Even if you do not know God I would have to ask, "What do you have to loose"? Are you willing to leave any possible help for your child off the table just because YOU do not believe? What if all you had to do was reach out to God for the sake of your child? Is that so hard to do? Prayer is a powerful tool that at the very least gives your child hope that there is something bigger than them, you or the doctors that may help them. As I said you and your child will need everything possible going for everyone involved to get through this. I even prayed for my doctors when I was going through my ordeal. You may be surprised at the outcome. I have found that these are the types of situations that help people discover the Lord and make the family even closer.

When you are with your child you must try to be yourself. Do not let your emotions dictate your behavior around them. You want things to seem as normal as possible for them. Stressed behavior and negative emotions will just find their way right to them and make them feel the same. Stress removes energy that they need to fight the disease. That is why I said I feel it is important to make sure they are as relaxed, happy and comfortable as possible. This will preserve energy that they may need to get through a treatment or tough situation. Believe me, after a while, all this adds up and it will make them weaker and weaker. They need to have all the strength mentally and physically they can get. Do not forget to take care of yourself through this also. It is necessary that they see you as strong and optimistic as possible. If they see hope in your eyes, it will make them hopeful. This will be physically draining for you also. Do not forget to make sure you are eating right, getting enough sleep and taking care of yourself medically also. Do not be too proud or afraid to ask to see a counselor if need be. A lot of the hospitals offer counseling in conjunction with their child's treatment program. If you are unable to afford this financially, which paying for cancer treatment seems to do to a lot of people, there are many free counseling programs out there. Sometimes group therapy is great and makes one feel not so all alone. This may also give you an opportunity to gain strength through others.

I would also think if you know someone who has a child who has had Cancer and is doing very well, it may be a very positive thing for your child to meet them and interact with them, a little group therapy of their own so to say. Sometimes seeing that someone else their own age has fought through all this can have a very positive affect on a child. I am sure that another child will have a unique perspective on all this that may be something only the children understand. They may better communicate things to your child since they all speak the same language if you know what I mean. Someone to play with who understands may do much to achieve the goals I mentioned above. It will help them take their mind off their problems and enjoy life for a little while. Let them be themselves as only a child can be. Do not be too serious and overbearing. Seeing you in a state of heightened concern constantly will only alarm them and cause them to worry also. So much of this is emotional for both the child and the parent. We are human beings and emotions are part of our lives but it is imperative that the emotions you show around them are optimistic, joyful and full of hope. They and you must NEVER give up hope! Being in the hospital is also very lonely. Make sure they are seeing as many people as possible. Make sure their brothers and sisters are visiting often. Make sure to coach the child's brothers and sisters on how to conduct themselves when around the child. This may be incredibly difficult as children have a hard time controlling their emotions. Take some of their friends up to see them. Ask your family to go and see them, especially if they have a special affection for some of the family members such as Grandpa and Grandma or a favorite Uncle or Aunt. But I would make sure they understand what I have discussed so far about not being negative around them.

Another thing you as a parent of a child with Cancer should understand is that children do not possess the courage and strength of will that we as adults have. They will need you to help them keep the courage and will to live alive sometimes. If a child's prognosis seems to indicate that their Cancer will be a long term or continuing for some time to come your own strength of will may be tested. Concentrate on how precious your child is to you. Love is an emotion that can leap almost all hurdles in life. It can be one of the most powerful motivators there is for you and your child. You must remain patient. I know I am making this all sound so easy but these are things you can do to help your child survive or at least live longer. As someone who has had Cancer, I understand that just because my Cancer is not able to be detected by our current technology does not mean it will not come back. I must say though, I am extremely optimistic about the advances being made in the treatment of Cancer. The engineering of genomes and cells is making remarkable advances in the treatment of Cancer and many other diseases. This should be something you share with your child also. I would make sure the Oncologist is relaying this to your child also. The child will perceive it as more authentic and knowledgeable coming from the doctor. You know kids think everything mom and dad say has some motive or trick behind it to make them do something. Make sure their siblings know this too. They can encourage the child in a way no adult can.

It is so important to communicate with your child's Oncologist. Do as much research as you can and stay current on what is happening in the field of Oncology. For the sake of your child you must bear a great deal of the burden here and need to exhibit an optimistic, positive and happy atmosphere for your child. Even though they are young and do not understand fully what is happening they are very perceptive of emotion. My heart goes out to everyone who has a child with Cancer. I have seen the commercials on television hundreds of time and I still cry every time I see them. I pray for them every time I see the commercials. I encourage you to sincerely pursue the spiritual aspect of healing as I did. My prayers were answered and I believe with all my heart yours will be too in some way shape or form. Pray with your child as often as you can without depressing them. They are smart enough to sense when things are dire and they need you to help keep them strong. Make sure your prayers do not reflect that the end is near or things are in a dire state so to say. I cannot say God will save everyone's child if they pray but I know if you do not ask you may have no chance at all of getting his help. As I said before, I know if it were my child I would be pursuing any and all ways to heal them no matter what I thought. I will pray for your children. Stay strong!

CHAPTER XV

Spirituality and Phylosophy

I suppose some of you may be asking what these next two chapters have to do with Cancer. As you can see, I believe that there is definitely a spiritual aspect to healing. I believe that it important for people to understand how I view spirituality and theology and used it to help me with my healing. I also feel that how you view life from a philosophical aspect affects your inner self so to say and helps to maximize your mental attitude towards your healing. They say God uses adversity to build strength and character. I guess that means whatever his plan is for me, it must be a real doozy. I have now had fourteen major surgeries in my life with twelve related to Cancer. Eleven of those were in a six year period. As I have sat and proofread this material, I guess I had never thought about it all at one time before. The VA health care system lists twenty three current or past major illnesses for me. I cannot help but feel that God must love me so much. How could I not be here without God's help? Even those of you who are skeptical about God have to ask yourself a few questions at some point as you have read this book. I know only one thing, I am still alive. It also makes me ponder a story from the bible. Even though my knowledge of the bible is somewhat limited compared to many, this story was one I read in the past for some reason. More coincidence I guess. It is the story of the Book of JOB. For those of you that are not familiar with it, I will make it short.

Job was a man who had great faith in God. He often talked to

God during his day. He had a wonderful wife and many wonderful children. He had a fishing fleet and a very nice home. In other words he had it all. He was living large as we say these days. One day God and Satan were talking and God was showing Satan the faith that Job had in him (God). The devil replied that of course Job did. He had everything a man could want in life and had no reason not to be faithful. He then told God that if Job were to lose everything he would turn on the Lord and curse him. The Lord said that Job's faith was too great. The devil smirked. So God told the devil he could have him(Job) but he could not kill him. Satan then took everything from Job. Killed off his family, took his health and all his worldly belongings. Even though Job asked God why this was happening to him, he never lost faith in God. Are you seeing any parallels here? I have lost my health, home, marriage, business and everything but my children. I do not profess to be anything like Job but it does go to attest to what can happen if you have faith in God and try to live a good life and love your fellow man. I have my own reasons as to why I believe this has happened to me. I have seen with my own eyes what faith has brought me. I will never lose faith in God. By the way, when Job's ordeal was over, he was rewarded seven fold by God!

Today I live in my little apartment and am not concerned with the things in life I used to. I live on a very modest income that is provided to me by the Veteran's Administration, a few SNAP benefits and my free phone. As a matter of fact, a short time ago I blew the engine in my car and had no idea what I was going to do. I certainly did not have the two thousand plus dollars I needed to have it fixed. But as with Job, I did not lose the faith. I was walking to get where I needed to go and my daughter helped with transportation if I needed to get me around for shopping and the like. It was very hard to walk with my COPD and if it was hot and humid, it was torture. One day I was walking over to the library as I did not have Internet and they have free access there. About half way there I had to stop. I was bent over and obviously struggling to catch my breath. As I was stopped, my mechanic just happened to drive by and he saw me. He later told me he had tried to stop but traffic would not allow it. The next day

I got a call from my daughter and she told me to call my mechanic. She said he had tried to call me but I was out of minutes so the call did not come to me.

Guess what, he had a car and was going to give it to me. One of his customers had decided not to pay for a car he had made repairs on. He had told my mechanic to keep the car and sell it to pay for the repairs he had done. He told me we could just swap the title of my now no good car for his now good running car. Not only had he made the repairs that the previous owner had needed, but made sure everything else on the vehicle was in good running order. I was shocked and did not know what to say. Again I cried. His act showed so much kindness by one person to another. He could have sold that car and got his money back. But instead he saw me and extended a hand of kindness. I thanked God and asked him to bless my mechanic for what he had done. This was no small thing he had done for me in my eyes. The pain and suffering of walking would now be gone. He was certainly an example of man at his best. Kindness and love for thy fellow man is not dead after all in this world. I know, another coincidence. To you I can only say to, REALLY?

I am not able to understand why God is doing this. I just know he is and I am thankful. I mean after all, who better to understand evil and overcome it, than he who has been at the bottom of the pit. I have told him repeatedly, anything you need Lord. I have begged to return the favor so to say. I do realize he has a sense of humor. Life is not all about Sin and all that you know. I was also trying to go to church again for a while but it did not take me long to figure out that it was not the church for me.

I tried to do fellowship, but almost everything coming out of people's mouths sounded like a tape recording of the bible. They spoke nothing from the heart or any real wisdom from God. They offered nothing inspiring, just a lot of repeated words. I do believe that if you have this disease, and you reach out to God, he CAN help you if HE chooses to. I certainly do not know who is and is not worthy of his help but I do believe that if you reach out sincerely and do right by him, he will help. It does not take a brilliant person to figure out that you will never find an egg if you do not go to the Easter Egg Hunt! If you do not reach out, I seriously doubt anything will change. There are those who do not bother because they think they have done things that have made them unworthy in his eyes. Let me tell you, no one is more unworthy than me and look where I am. He is forgiving of those who realize their mistakes and are truly sorry for having made them. Just ask and I bet he will show you that he does forgive. Let me say it this way. Do you not forgive your children when they do something wrong? Why? Because you love them and you know that they are children and this is part of the learning process of growing up to adulthood. Are we not the children of God? Then I would say the same thing applies to you. I will say though, your repentance better come from the heart. Do not think that you will fool him with your words, remember who and what he is.

I called this book what I did because I believe each of us has a little piece of God in us. That is our spirit. That spirit lives in our physical body while we are alive on this earth for a period of time. What we do here affects what that spirit becomes and is at the time of our passing. That time when our physical body ceases to exist and that spirit moves on. Where it goes and what happens to it is determined by what we do during our time here. Life is a precious gift and should not be wasted. I would ask you, if someone gave you a wonderful gift, something you had always wanted, would you not cherish it? What if you treated that present badly or ruined it needlessly, do you think they would ever give you another present? He gave you a life on earth and if you use it for wrong, he will not give you that present of the next life. When I was in the hospital, sometimes I would go to the Oncology wards and see people who had been diagnosed with Cancer. It seemed like so many cried and were feeling sorry for themselves. I would be willing to bet, those people would go home and lie on the couch and wait to die. Why when we are getting so close to curing so many types of Cancer? God gave us many ways to help ourselves. Faith, family, medicine and just plain old fortitude are but a few. You must fight to keep your present that

God gave you. Enjoy what time you have left. I love you and want to see you where the next place is.

After I had my resection done, our family went to Myrtle Beach on vacation. I was in so much pain and feeling sorry for myself. I soon realized I was focused on all the wrong things. I watched my children laughing and having fun and before I realized it, I was laughing with them and having fun too. You can go through life being happy or sad, the choice is yours. But only you can make the choice. I hope people will read this book and realize that. If I help some people live longer and be happier, then my work will not have been in vain. Cancer is most often a long, slow and progressive disease that devastates everyone around it. I have watched people who find out they have Cancer and give up shortly after they get the news. It is sad, they always seem to be the ones that die first. I had a neighbor who had Liver Cancer and was told he only had six months to live. He told them what they could do with their six months. He fought and called on God to help as I have. He did die of Liver Cancer, NINE YEARS later! And what kind of doctor tells his patient that they only have so much time to live? Talk about an insurance policy for death! Your doctor is not God, he can estimate, but that is all. Most likely, he does not know your strengths and weakness.

If you have a family member or loved one with this horrible disease, give them all the spiritual, emotional financial or any other type of help you can. I truly believe that there are spiritual and mental components to healing that are just as or maybe even more important than on the medical side. As I am sitting here in the hospital writing, one of my doctors came in and was impressed with my writings. He is from China. Healing is much different there. He proceeded to tell me about a study just published by a Purdue University doctor seemed to indicate what I have just said is true. It proved your mental strength, attitude and frame of mind are just as important as everything else. If you have faith in God, Love of Family, and the proper frame of mind, YOU WILL LIVE LONGER! I must also mention another weird coincidence has occurred as he was walking into the room. My next sentence as I was typing was going to be, "I do not know for sure, but I am sure someone had done a study proving this...." Is someone trying to tell me something or what?

This can be a tough job though. One must search one's soul and come to certain realizations. We are after all, human, as the saying goes. You must first be willing to search for truth objectively with an open mind. This becomes more difficult as we age. We become set in out ways. Our experiences in life tend to set a template for our beliefs and understanding. It is difficult to change and be objective due to those experiences and how we perceived those events that took place in our lives. They are the basis for how we think and respond to all that takes place in our lives. How we see ourselves and others. It forms a basis for how we assess and make judgments. How we will do things. It all requires some pretty serious thinking and contemplation. And you can bet that huge pit-fall called self-pity will cloud our judgment of things and cause us to fall prey to Satan.

As a species we are definitely going in the toilet so to say. We are lazy and materialistic. Attributes such as ambition and pride in our accomplishments seem to be more and more a thing of the past. Addicted to our electronics and our "stuff". Caught up in a rat race that seems to be leading us to corruption, greed, turmoil and violence. A lot of people are fearful of the future. In a strange sort of way, we are trading our integrity, honesty and our spirits for ease, convenience and the material things in life. Things that used to be rock solid attributes and a gauge of who and what one was are becoming a thing of the past. Flowing away as the next group of politicians, lawmakers and profit takers come to power. The law is a joke that no longer has meaning grounded in solid principals. It now means whatever those in power want it to mean according to whichever way the winds are blowing today. Why do you think so many are trying so hard to rid our society and government of God. When God is gone, those in power will decide what is right and what is wrong. It will not take long for good people to realize that they are the losers in this type of society. The problem is, at that point it will be too late for our species. Satan will have won.

There was once a man named Edmund Burke who put it quite

succinctly. He said, "The only thing necessary for the triumph of evil is for good men to do nothing". I believe if you read Revelations in the Bible, you will find that some of what it says seems to be coming to fruition right before our very eyes. I do not claim to be a student of the Bible that some people are, but I do have enough common sense to see what is happening around me. By the way, common sense is not so common any more. People are being browbeaten by government, media, corporations and even their own peers into perceiving the world as something the world is not. It talks in Revelations about everything becoming an "Illusion". Take advertising for instance. Why do we need the nearly invisible "disclaimers" at the bottom of the ads we see every day? It is because if companies told you the truth you would never buy their goods and services. Why can they not just make a good product with quality features and be done with it? God's laws never change and are not deceptive. You know what you are getting right up front and he always stands behind his words. Our laws are written by everyone except the people who are supposed to write them. Lobbyists and financial influences are the primary force behind the crafting of our laws now. God's laws have been here forever and have never changed in all the time that man has been here on this earth. I think that is the true definition of "Rock Solid".

Even though technology and the things of this earth have changed, we as a species still have the same two basic needs we did when God put us here. Those are the need for food and shelter. Everything after that is a choice and the world and its people seem to be making a lot of BAD choices. Look at all the churches that are more concerned about their money and their 501C3 exemption status than they are about doing the Lord's work. The service opens with discussions about money and events that have no bearing on the spiritual lives of the parishioners. Everyone comes to the service like good little boys and girls and then go out and do things all week that I sure God would frown on or even make him downright angry. Look at all the Mega churches that exist today. Have you ever noticed how well off the people that run the joint are? They pretend to live the life of holier than thou. I will never forget a story my wife told me about a pastor at one of the largest churches in our city. She was a waitress at one of the local restaurants. She told me a story about a pastor of what is probably the largest church in our area. He would come in with his mistress before services every Sunday. They would sit in one of the back booths and smooch and giggle. Then after church he would come in with his wife and family. And believe me this family that ran this church was worth millions! And I am sure this is not the exception to the rule in today's world.

God also says he will keep things simple. He does not want your rituals and traditions. He wants what is in YOUR heart. He wants what is genuinely you. Not the rituals someone in the church tells us to believe and practice. We justify our sins in our minds and feel better for having done it afterwards. It's all about the "feelings" these days. What our intentions are and not the results. Imagine going into court and say, "But your honor I did not MEAN to murder him". The fact that you took a life is not supposed to matter if you did not "mean" to do it. Yet that seems to be the direction our world is heading. No accountability for our actions. I think to God, your actions speak louder than your words. Not to say God does not tolerate failure. I believe he just wants you to give your very best. If you fail he will forgive you. You are after all, human. Revelations also speaks of a mirroring of the world. Right and good will become bad and wrong and vice versa. Why does it seem that for so many people Satan is winning this game we are calling life? Look at Jesus and the story of his life. He ran into opposition everywhere he went. Yet he stood steadfast in his beliefs even as they were pounding the nails into his body. He even begged God, his father, to forgive the men who were doing this to him!

We are being told we need to be a diverse society and be tolerant of others. I believe what is being passed off as "Law" is just a bunch of legislative gobaldygoop. Political Correctness run amuck. It could all be replaced with just two words, fairness and honesty. People have become irresponsible in their own affairs and responsibilities in the name of convenience. They claim they do not have the time yet they spend hours on their computers and phones absorbed in the social media craze. We seem to have more excuses these days than Quaker has oats. We trust many of the aspects of our lives to people who have not earned that trust. Take buying a car for instance. People sit down to close the deal on the car and sign a three page legal document that they do not understand. All they know is that they sign and get to leave with their new car. There was a time when a man would never sign his name to something he did not understand. Look at the "Affordable Care Act". When it came time for the Congress to vote on it, they were told by the Speaker of the House, "You will have to vote on it to find out what is in it". And instead of telling her where to put that Act of Congress, they did exactly that, they voted for it and passed it. How irresponsible is that? It has now become a source of great turmoil and division in our country. An Act of Congress pushed upon the people of this country by people with ideals of power and personal legacy.

It has taken me a long time to realize and understand that none of this is really that important. We are on this earth but a moment and it is what comes after that is important. I have felt a physical presence in my body before that I have no doubt was divine in its nature. Some of you will think what you will, but if you take the time to search openly and objectively, you will be surprised at what you will find. No self-justification, interpretation or lying to yourself. What do you have to lose? That old life will still be there when you finish your quest. But maybe, just maybe, you will discover something new. You just may discover a new life and a new way of thinking and living. As for those of you who do not believe anything that is not tangible to one or more of your physical senses, I feel sorry for you and will pray for you. You are going to miss so much. Everything in your life has some connection to this earth. I used to think that way. The only thing is you start to long for something more out of life. Sooner or later you are going to ask yourself the question, "Is this all that I am? Is this all that life is?"

We are not just the physical being that we all know so well. That spirit lives within us and it needs to be nurtured to grow and reach that next plane. I am trying to make that spiritual being the most important thing in my life right now. I have spent my entire life wasting this gift of life God gave me. I know now he has laid out a different path for me to follow. I believe with all my heart, God had something he wants me to do. He has not saved me for no reason. I do not have any idea what that thing is, but when he calls, I will answer. I hope whatever it is, I can do it well for him. I hope someday to be worthy of his praise. I am passionate about helping people and finding out what he has in store for me next. God Bless You all!

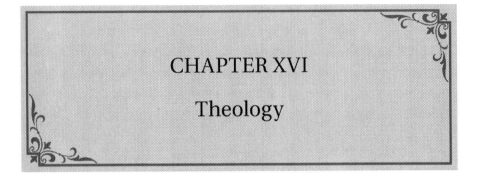

CHAPTER XVI

Theology

I would like to start this chapter saying that I make no claims to being some type of omnipotent man who knows all or thinks he does anyways. Most of what I have written is based on my opinion or experiences in life. It is how I observe the world through MY eyes. I am sure that this chapter will offend some of you. I am sure some will say I am an arrogant this or that. I will say also that if this chapter offends you, maybe you might want to take a long look at yourself with honest and objective criticism. I would also like to say, that in my eyes, there is a difference between "Religion" and "Spirituality". I also do not confuse "Religions" with "Faiths". I have come to realize there are way too many "Experts" when it comes to Theology. By the way, an "Ex" is a has been, and a "Spert" is a drip under pressure. Put them both together and what have you got? Remember, we have to keep that sense of humor.

It is easy to differentiate between the spiritual and the religious. I love it when someone who says they are a spiritual person asks me if I "Believe" in God. This would seem to imply that you have a choice, almost like whether to have waffles or eggs for breakfast. God is not someone you believe in, he is someone you know. Do you "believe" your next door neighbor lives there, or do you "Know" he does. Once you have seen him walk into his house, you know he lives there. The same as it is with God. Once you discover his existence you do not believe in him, you know him! I am always reluctant to use the words someone or something in reference to the Lord. But for the ease of writing and as a reference point for us in our own minds, I will say he or someone. I also hear those same people refer to a relationship with God. How can you have a relationship with someone if you do not "Know" them?

The religious use the Bible to substantiate their opinions and feelings and are usually doing most of the talking. If you listen carefully, you will find the words they use are not theirs, but words they have memorized from the Bible or that of a man they call their spiritual leader. People who are truly spiritual also listen and exchange ideas that consist of words that come from their heart. I believe it is referred to as "Fellowship". Ever notice how some people seem to be able to pull scripture out of the air like a rabbit out of a hat at a magic show to substantiate just about any point of view they have? I understand that a great many people read the Bible and have memorized a great deal of it. My question is, do they understand what they are reading without someone else translating it for them? I do not trust man or his motives when it comes to God and his word. Remember, Satan is "The Great Deceiver"! The Bible was written centuries before anyone on this earth now was born and has been translated many times and many ways by "Men". I am sure that there are those who will say that those men were "Inspired" by God or "Guided" by God or something of that nature.

I will give you an example of the type of changes men make to the Bible and its teachings. Again, I do not claim to be an authority on the subject, but I do know a few things. I am sure most of you have read the Ten Commandments at some time in your life. One of the commandments most people have been taught is the one that says "Thou shalt not kill". Well I got news for you folks, someone changed that somewhere along the way because what it actually says is, "Thou shalt not Murder". Now some of you may ask what the difference is and to you I say go buy a dictionary and find out. To me that is no subtle change. It also makes me wonder what other subtle or not so subtle changes have been made by men along the way to give us what we have today.

Most of the Bible was written in Biblical Hebrew with some portions written in Biblical Aramaic. The very first translations were from the Biblical Hebrew to Greek. They were written on parchment that has deteriorated over the centuries. If you know anything about man's greedy and corrupted history, you know how many doors all this opens to interpretation and plain old "filling in the gaps" all this brings. Take the "King James" version of the Bible. It is probably the most widely read of the Bibles in existence. The writing of this Bible was controlled and supervised by King James and was completed in 1611. Now knowing what we know about those times and the men who ruled, do you not think good old King James made sure that what appeared in that writing was what HE wanted it to be? As a man, do you think it is possible he could have had any ulterior motives or influences on those writings? Just think of how much of our current history is being rewritten for the sake of "Political Correctness" and ideals that are not a true reflection if history. Do you not think powerful men with motives other than God's could not have, over time, made those changes for their own gain?

Time changes all things. Even the present day media realizes that most people forget what they told them two weeks ago and use that memory lapse and uncertainty to their advantage. I think that many "Religious" people consider their "expertise" on the words in the Bible as being spiritual. They seem to think that is what God wants them to do. How many of them are simply driven by pride because they think that is what God wants them to do. By the way, "Pride" is a sin. These people speak of fishing for men. I am not sure what they are fishing for, but I seriously doubt they are saving a lot of souls. Yes we should all know the history, lessons and wisdom taught to us by the Bible but it is not the only source of wisdom and the teachings of God on this earth. Do you think God put all this here for us to ignore and spend all our time learning and contemplating the words of the Bible? And for that matter, lighten up folks. Sin and discipline are not the only lessons here to be taught. How about forgiveness, joy and all of the wonders of this earth? Are these things not all great gifts from God for us to learn from? Are there not lessons to be learned with our eyes and ears? This earth has great beauty and many wonders on it that we also may learn from. Not to mention learning from each other and our experiences in life. So get your head out of that Bible and live a little. Can we not walk and chew bubble gum at the same time?

Many people attend Bible studies and fellowship meetings where someone else does most of the talking or tells them THEY are wrong in how they perceive God and his wonders. I have told my children to listen to their hearts. To listen to that inner voice, or that gut feeling as some like to call it. A spiritual person listens to others also and understands that many points of view are needed to make one a well-rounded person. If what you hear is not righteous, your heart will tell you. We have that thing in us called conscience. Your spirit tells you what is right and wrong. You may not pay attention to it or heed its warnings, but it is there. It seems to be getting harder and harder to decipher through all the garbage that is called news and information that is out there in our world today. Finding truth can be a challenge. There is so much deception coming at us from every angle it can hard to stay true to God. I feel this is just another way that Satan deceives and distracts us from what is really important. He lays power, money and the material things at our feet to claim as our own. God owns EVERYTHING! Satan gets us to trade our souls for the things of this world. Greed is one of his most powerful tools. I have known some very wealthy people in my life. Most of them treasured there "Stuff" more than anything. They are also usually willing to sacrifice anything to keep it too.

I have been to twenty eight countries and major island chains during my life. I have seen many different faiths, religions and cultures and they all seem to have one thing in common, a God. I find it odd that so many people kill each other in the name of God. What kind of God tells men to kill innocent men, women and children in its name? I used the term "it's name" there because whatever god tells us to kill innocent people is not the real God. That kind of god IS an IT! Every religion seems to think THEIR way is the ONLY way. Some religions think all others must die except the people of their religion. War in the name of God has never made much sense to me. Rage seems to be everywhere these days. We used to know how to relax and enjoy the true comforts of life. Now everyone is going Mach two with their hair on fire to obtain more "stuff" or to find the ultimate thrill. And we cannot figure out why our children are such a mess and we are exhausted all the time? Settle down folks, Instagram and Facebook will be there when you get back. Our kids are a mess because so many parents know nothing about parenting and even less, if anything, about God and spirituality. It is the most massive case of the blind leading the blind in history. Look around and see how many people are addicted to their phones, computer and pads. Watch as people drive by and see how many have a phone to their ears. Who do all these people talk to all the time? Yet as I said before, we just do not have the time to do what is right in this world. I would say we have a very screwed up sense of priorities.

I also believe it is going to get a whole lot worse before it gets better. I see war coming. First I see a war between men over power, material things and earthly beliefs. Then, when that war is over, I see a war between spiritual men and Satan and his minions. I do not pretend to know when, but they are coming. I sometimes get very strange looks from those who believe themselves to be spiritual people. When I disagree with them and I explain why I feel the way I do, they get angry and question MY spirituality. They try to discredit me with scripture from the bible that they pull out of the air to substantiate their point of view. What makes them all knowing, all seeing people with some special insight to what God wants us to do? Are they not men just like me? Do they possess some special qualification given to them by God that I cannot see or understand? Maybe some do, but I doubt that most do. There always seems to be a condescending nature about them as if they are better than me or something.

We have seen the decline of our morals little by little. Even in my short time on this earth things have changed dramatically. I remember when I was young and one night we went to the drive-in movies. The last movie of the evening was a James Bond movie. My parents made all of us children lay down in the back of the car and go to sleep. We were not allowed to see such "adult" movies. Such things were considered very risqué and not for children. Today our children turn on the television or computer and see anything they want. I guess that is what scares me. The progression of the evil is getting faster and faster and there seems to be very little resistance to it by society. Just about anything seems to be alright. I am not so naive as to believe that some of these things have not been here as long as man has. Adultery and prostitution are two of our oldest sins. But at least in the past they seemed to be thought of as evil and were confined to dark places. Now everything is everywhere and no one seems to care. Especially if it is something government wants or companies profit from.

Some of you will say nothing is really different now than in the past. That it is just more noticeable and widely seen due to the technology we have now. Well to me, more widely seen means an expansion of evil if more people are seeing and experiencing it! And it also means it is more likely to be accepted by society. At the time of this writing the atrocities of Nice, France and Orlando Florida had just happened. I have been telling people for years that the people of the Middle East would not take our interference in their affairs lightly. I pointed out what the Israelis were experiencing and said that someday that will be us. People thought I was nuts. "Not here, this is the United States of big bad America", they would say. Look at us now.

Satan whittles away at our righteousness a little at a time. Carving away at it sliver by sliver. He realizes if you make to drastic a change too quickly, people will notice. He knows if you make small gradual changes over a long period of time, people will not notice and are much less likely to offer any resistance to such changes. Some may even say something stupid like, "That's progress". Before you know it, we have gone from A to Z and did not even realize it has happened. We are mortal, Satan is not. He knows every generation will forget or change history to suit their needs. Time is on his side and time forgets all things. I find it interesting that so many people just roll over and play dead to whatever government, corporations and other people tell them or others to do. We have become comfortable, complacent and lazy. Incapable of independent thought. We seem to have lost all will when it comes to what is really important yet we are willing to put forth great effort to fight and argue over the trivial things. We have become petty and inconsiderate of our fellow man. Anger is a vicious circle as Satan knows so well. He uses the tools of this earth and our emotions against us to reach his goals for us. Our frustrations and dislikes. Our impatience and desire for instant gratification. And, as the title of this book implies, illness and disease. We are an overly emotional species these days exercising a great deal of bad judgment. It seems so much of what we do leads to the wasting of resources such as ourselves and our planet. Look at the garbage generated by mankind in a single day. And all that came from the resources God put here for us. Satan will use any form of negativity against us to take dominion over those spirits residing inside of us we call our souls.

Do you not find it strange that we have so many documents, including our fake money, that have some reference to God on them, yet the government says it cannot have anything to do with God. Do you really think that our founding fathers really meant for us to live a life free of spirituality. A world where we turn on the God switch in our private lives but are told to turn it off when it comes to government and our public lives? Are they suggesting that we can only be spiritual on a part time basis? I would say to you, God does not want any part timers! Our spirit is inherent within us and no government can take it away from us or tell it what to do.

Our spirituality is the basis for our very existence. Did you know that the so called "Separation of Church and State" clause we hear touted so much by people in government is actually nowhere in the Constitution of our great country? They are words from a court decision. Words of a man called a Judge. What was it God said about the Judges? We cannot leave our spirituality and beliefs at the door when we leave our homes. I think that scares Satan and his earthly minions too. If there is one thing those in power realize is the fact that there is power in numbers. I often wonder if and how long it will take before things become so unbearable for people that they finally do something. It is funny how the government bends over backwards to defend the rights of the greedy and non-spiritual at the expense of these who do know God and live by his teachings. Are we who know God not having our "Unalienable God given rights" taken away by making us live our lives this way? Where are the defenders of OUR rights? It is just another level of control for them. Where is the government President Lincoln spoke of at Gettysburg where he talked about a government "Of the people, by the people and for the people"? The problem is the people have stopped participating. A great many people have died for those ideals yet we are watching those ideals slowly slip away and doing nothing to stop it. Living in our own little worlds obsessed with ourselves and our "Stuff". What a shame.

Have you noticed how many laws we have nowadays? These are the laws of men and not of God. I seriously doubt most people realize it, but most of our laws are not really "Laws". They are statutes. If we continue to make laws about petty things such as "Hate Crimes", it will not be long before you will not be able to live your life without breaking some law. So when they come for you, do not complain. Your inaction all these years is bringing us to a point where we will all be doomed. You will be subjects of a government of men who care about nothing but their own ambitions, money and power. People really need to pay attention to what is happening to our language too. Words are powerful and Satan knows this. They affect how we think about things and perceive them. Why do you think that those in power have controlled the institutions of the media since the beginning of time? Control what and how information is presented to the masses and you will control their thinking. Rules and laws were created to protect us and give structure and organization to our lives. Look at the rules and laws of today. Are they accomplishing that? I think they are being used to control and manage us at the expense of our freedoms, one of which is our ability to use our judgment to make decisions.

Judgment is a critical part of our existence. We judge, or choose, which cleaner is better than another. We judge, or choose, who to vote for and so on. Rules and laws are being created that are taking our ability to "choose" away from us. That is just another method of establishing control. How many times are we being told to be "Diverse" and not "Judge" people or judge something? Then you are told you are a bad person if you do. If you are a somewhat intelligent person, you realize we are constantly judging many things in our lives. Judgment is at the end of a process we call evaluation. How are we to know if someone or something is good or bad if we do not evaluate and use judgment in our lives? How will we know what is right and wrong? This is just another way for the evil to continue. They want you to let them tell you what is good and what is bad. They will tell you how and what to decide. Satan sits and laughs at us and our pettiness and self-absorbed stupidity.

Do you see the connection? If you are made to believe that judgment is bad, you will stop evaluating and you will need someone else's (government's or some corporation's) help to make decisions about your life. More control. The big question is who is controlling them? I have been able to come to only one conclusion, Satan! There are a great many people in our world making a living from all this turmoil. Open your phone book to the yellow pages and see how many lawyers are listed. I bet they take up a third or a fourth of the listings there. Satan also keeps us divided. He divides our faiths, races and classes, to name but a few. Too many are being manipulated for gain by others. I do not wish anyone to believe that I am anti-government or one of those other names they use to demonize people who think as I do and do not play their game. Any intelligent individual realizes that we must have government to do a great many things in this world. Yet we see so much turmoil, death and destruction that are the direct result of government.

Earlier in this book I made a statement about choice. I cannot help but wonder why man has made so many BAD and destructive choices. I am but a man myself so I do not know the answer, but I would sure like to know. It seems that for so many, that dark side that comes from Satan seems to attract more people for some reason. Maybe someday God will enlighten me. See what the lack of a good and righteous sense of judgment does to us and wonder what God thinks about the fact that mankind has devoted more time, wealth, effort and lives to one thing more than any other. Something we all claim is so terrible. That one thing is WAR. Just think what our lives would be like if we had devoted all those things and resources to making our lives and world a better place. Where would medicine be today? Where would education and science be? I do not believe that God created this world and all its resources for us to use to kill each other and wage war. And the thing of it is we all know better!

God gave us a sense of judgment that is built in. It is called conscience. Just ask yourself before you do something, "Would I want that done to me?" I wonder how many of us would answer no and still do it? It seems fairness and honesty are quickly becoming a thing of the past. When you talk to people, are they direct and to the point? I have noticed people do not speak like they used to. I believe this is for two reasons. The first is because they may be afraid of offending someone. Ain't Political Correctness great? The other is that they are figuring out what to say and how to say it because they believe the answer they get will not be honest or truthful. Cynicism of each other seems to be rampant. No one trusts each other anymore. And I guess I must say, a lot of the time it is with good cause. This covers anything from a little white lie to the boldest lies ever told and anything in between. It seems that so many people have an angle or agenda these days. We are cynical and deceptive. We feel we must protect ourselves from others who are basically doing the same thing we are. What a vicious circle!

I cannot help but wonder what God thinks of his creation. Is he sad that so many of us are a disappointment. Does he say, "I gave them a chance and they blew it? "I gave them everything the needed to make the world a wonderful and magnificent place". Instead they were selfish and greedy so they will get what they deserve. I want to reach as many people as possible with these words. I also believe that no matter what your faith is or who you call God, he will be forgiving if you try to set things right. It only makes sense that God being omnipotent, would know ahead of time that many of us would mess up this wonderful gift we call life. He knew we were "human". I also believe that he has given us all a way to repent and realize what he hoped for us. For example, for Christians, Jesus is their way to salvation. I am not familiar enough with other religions to know what their way to salvation is, but I know that way is there for them too. Yet again, division is created. The division between the different beliefs and faiths of this earth. Do Christians believe that they are the only ones who will go to heaven? I have traveled to many places on this earth and met many fine and spiritual people of different faiths that were not Christians. I believe men have different paths. God is good and evil is evil, no matter what your faith or what path that faith takes to ascend to that place we commonly call heaven. I believe we as men need much of this as a reference point because of the limitations placed upon us by our corporeal existence and our own feeble brains.

As I said before, I do not mean to sound like I know everything. I am really just hoping to get you to thinking. Much is opinion and some is conjecture. I often wonder what doors open if we are one of the lucky ones who make it to whatever comes after our mortal life on this earth. Will all of my questions be answered? I have a lot of questions I would love to have answered. It seems to me, the way we think as human beings or at least a large portion of our thoughts will be totally irrelevant once we transcend from our corporeal bodies to that of being in a totally spiritual state. I am not really sure what that state of being is, but knowing God, I bet it is really something. As people of this earth, we can only imagine and I bet that does not even come close. I am amazed at our arrogance as a race of beings. We think we are so smart but in actuality, we know so little. We cannot even travel to the next little body in the sky we call the moon without a major effort by thousands of people.

Our world today is changing at an astonishing rate. As I have said before, I am not that old but one thing I have noticed is the amount of change is increasing and the speed at which it is changing is increasing too. In our fast paced world, a lot of attention to detail is being cast aside. In the end, that will lead to sloppiness in our own lives and the affairs of the world. The family structure is falling by the wayside. I heard a statistic the other day that just floored me. Even if it is remotely close to accurate, it speaks to a lot of why we are in so much trouble. A study had been done on the number of children born out of wedlock (no fathers) by race as a percentage. The statistics were as follows: Blacks-73%, Hispanics-52% and Caucasians-28%. I guess they did not think about the Orientals. I was amazed! And we cannot figure out why our world is so crazy? Do people not realize that men and women are very different and both contribute many of the things that are extremely significant to the raising of a child? Many of those things are unique to their sex. Children need both to grow up as well rounded individuals with a sense of understanding of both men and women. Both have a unique perspective that only a person of their sex is able to offer.

Have you noticed how little marriage seems to mean these days. Our commitment to our spouse seems to be as throw away as our society. The words "I'm sorry" seem to come a bit too easy these days and just do not have the tone of sincerity they used to have. If I hear the term "My Bad" one more time I think I am going to scream.

CHAPTER XVII

Find Your Strength

Now that you have heard my story can you start to see some of the changes you will have to make to improve your life and the lives of those around you? Your illness IS a battle and you must decide if you are going to WIN it or lose it. It is up to you. As I said before, I am only a human being just like you. I found my strengths in God and anywhere else I could draw them from. He and others have helped me to reach deep within myself and find enormous strength I never knew I had. You must be righteous and give your spirit to the Lord in return for his help. You must give it sincerely and from the heart. GOD WANTS YOU! Can you not see what you are capable of if you really try? Be strong and unwavering in your relentless push to keep going and enjoy life. Consider the most precious things in life such as God, family and friends to draw strength from. They WILL get you through it. Will it be easy? Probably not, you have this terrible disease remember. You have the ability to find out what works for you and motivates you to keep on going. To find out what makes this life worth living and continuing. You will have to reach deep inside yourself and find what you need to keep going.

I will say I believe with all my heart that if you give up spiritually and mentally, you will die. Take hold of every beautiful moment you have left. These are the moments that make life worth living. I have Cancer and am going to "Die" just does not cut it folks. I have Cancer and I am going to "LIVE"! That is the message you must tell yourself.

Take advantage of every waking moment to live life to its fullest. No one knows when you are going to die except God. I just hate it when doctors try to tell patients they only have so much time to live. As I said before, that is an insurance policy for death. I would think that even those of you who are yet to discover your spirituality can see that science is making great strides in the field of Cancer research. So even from that frame of mind you would think you would want to try and hang on for as long as possible. Tomorrow may be your day! The day they find a cure for the type of Cancer YOU have. There is a disease called Hepatitis C that has killed a great many people over the years. I heard a statistic on television the other day that said that one out of ten baby boomers has this disease. Yet through the types of aforementioned research, there are now cures for this disease. These cures did not exist even ten years ago. I speak from personal experience concerning this topic. I also had this disease until recently. Now, due to the research and development of new types of drugs, I no longer have this disease. This was a disease that could very well have killed me someday. Recent Genome research is taking aim at a great many diseases. Hang in there, it may be your turn next!

You must learn to decipher through all the deceptive emotions that Satan uses against you such as hate, anger and despair to keep you from focusing on what is really needed for you to reach your maximum spiritual link to God and using it to heal yourself. Remember, Satan knows this earth will be returned to what God meant it to be some day and when that happens, he will be very angry and taking as many souls with him as he can. Remember the second war I spoke of earlier? Look at our children and all the horror, sex and violence being thrust upon them by the media, corporations, government and their peers. Everything is becoming a grey area where self-discipline and restraint are considered odd and old fashioned. They are too young to understand and develop good judgment in their lives. They are lost and with no one to turn to in many cases because their parents have never been taught themselves. So many parents are using what I call the "Buddy Experiment" in the raising of their children. You are not their "buddy" or "friend", you are their parent. They are being brought up in a world of disrespect, anger and no compassion or empathy for their fellow man. Living in a society that practices the doctrine of "get as much as you can with as little effort as possible".

One other emotion that I see to be prevalent among Cancer patients and I consider to be one of our greatest down falls is self-pity. Man did I live that one for a while. If you look objectively at yourself, are you guilty of this emotion? Are you using it as a way to deal with life and with your loved ones? It keeps us weak and distracted. We tell ourselves we have Cancer and our heads start spinning. We see the death and suffering this disease brings to so many and just tell ourselves that will be me some day. Being objective, I do believe that there is probably a direct relationship between the severity of the disease and the amount of self-pity we experience. Yet having said that, I still believe even the most severe stages of Cancer can be overcome with God's help and the right combination of powerful spiritual, medical and personal strengths that are available to us if we would just get out of bed and pursue them.

This also does not consider the selfishness we are exhibiting towards our families, friends and loved ones. Do you not think that you are extending your misery to all of them too? Do not forget the power of prayer from others! I have heard so many people tell me that they prayed for me during this time in my life. And I mean A LOT of people prayed for me. Just knowing that so many people cared enough to take the time to pray for me was a very humbling experience. I guess with the sins of my past, I could not understand why so many would pray for me. This is yet another place to draw strength from. People can be such wonderful sources of joy and healing. I am someone who loves people and all the wonders associated with them. Especially precious are the children. They are our most precious resource! Does a child's laughter not just make you feel good inside when you listen to it? Interact with them and laugh with them. Remove your mind from the misery for a while. Do you remember my story about me and my kids at Myrtle Beach?

You can go through life being happy or sad, the choice is yours.

I know I am making all this sound easy. I would imagine some of you are reading this and wondering what kind of fairy tale is this guy living? I can only say one thing to you. Look at MY results! I have also come to realize that once you start to live and think this way, it becomes easier and easier to do. You start to realize the contrast between where you WERE and where you ARE and it motivates you to continue your pursuit of life. Keep fighting!

CHAPTER XVIII

The Government and Corporate Affect

Again, I write this chapter with some reluctance. I hope to portray the connection these two entities have to your health. The government affects health care through regulation and law. Corporations affect it through the need for profit. Both involve a never ending web of greed, bureaucracy and regulation that stifles everything from research, treatments and the production of new drugs to help fight disease. A couple of examples of the kinds of organizations that exist with each of these are the American Medical Association (AMA) on the corporate side, and the Food and Drug Administration (FDA) on the government side. And these are but two of the many organizations who make everything involved with developing and producing a new drug to treat or cure a disease almost impossible. This is not to mention the affect that insurance companies are having on your health. I am sure almost everyone dealing with the nightmare of Cancer has a list of stories they can tell about their insurance company. A wonderful combination of Accountants and Doctors sitting somewhere far away making critical decisions about YOUR health based on "Statistics" that someone has gathered along the way.

And all this is the mess we now call health care. And the regulations imposed on companies by government can be absolutely ridiculous. And oh yes, we Americans ARE footing the bill for an awful lot of the research. I cannot imagine where we would be if we had devoted all the money we have spent on war to curing illness and disease. I also wonder what the Lord thinks about that. It is funny how close government and corporations have become. And what about lawyers and their effect on the cost of health care! Everyone suing everyone for anything they can get. I firmly believe that the whole corporate structure was created by men to deflect liability from themselves for their own incompetency, laziness and greed. When it comes to health care, the liabilities become enormous. People get MAD when their lives or health are on the line and they want restitution when things go wrong. Someone must pay!

Why do you think there are so many lawyers that specialize in health care related law suits? Just watch your television and see all the ads for them. There was a time when these types of lawyers were referred to as "Ambulance Chasers" and their activities were frowned on. Not any more, as I said just look at your television. There is money to be made you know! These clever men are just waiting to help you with your problems, for a healthy fee of course. I had a friend who graduated from the John Hopkins School of Law. He was so repelled by the whole legal system he never even took his bar exams. I am sure that you have heard the term "Licensed to Practice Law" before. Actually such a "License" does not exist. Lawyers join the bar of whatever state they "Practice" law in. They receive no licenses as the term truly applies. My friend told me a joke I will never forget. He asked me, "How do you know if a lawyer is lying?" I responded by asking him how and he said, "If his lips are moving!" So many laws and regulations and most written by the lawyers and lobbyists that represent the very corporations that our lawmakers are supposed to be protecting us from. The men and women who run these corporations that are associated with the field of medicine and big Pharma as it is now called, are no longer made to be personally accountable. They belong to an elite class of people who have power and money and are part of a system designed to deflect such problems away from them personally. And believe me, our children are taking note of this behavior and trying to copy it in their own lives and other ways. The corporate structure takes the fall while Mr. CEO walks away with millions.

In some cases, like the case of T.A.R.P., a government program designed to bail out a whole list of greedy and immoral people who had nothing but their own enrichment in mind. These are people who had no problem asking the government to bail them out at the expense of YOU and FUTURE generations. Money they did not have to work for, but the fruits of you and future generation's labor. Debts created long before they even existed on this planet. Debts that they will be made to pay for through taxation. What kind of system are we living in now? Do you think it is a coincidence that so many in the government are lawyers? Law is supposedly the basis for our civilized society they will tell you. What a joke it has all become.

During one of my law classes in college, I was given an assignment to write a thesis on a certain aspect of law and it was to be so many pages long and all that. The paper I submitted was only one statement long. I said, "When the Law ceases to be the Servant of Justice and becomes the Servant of the Men who make those Laws, we are all doomed". I got an A. I was very young at that point in my life but my professor called me up to hand me my paper and told me what an astute young man I was for my age. Well I do not know about all that, but I was not so stupid that I could not see what was happening in the world around me! That is what slays me about it all. They do it right under our very noses under this pretense or that and we know it all stinks. Yet we just continue to stand idly by and watch it all happen. Whatever happened to the type of spirit that the men who formed this great county had? Willing to die for the principals that this great country was founded upon? We have become so accustomed to it we just trod along through life existing in our own little world and as long as there are no waves in it. We do not seem to care about what happens outside our little protective bubble.

We should all be ashamed. Many men have died so that we may have those principals and freedoms. Not anymore. They die for Oil and the spreading of "Democracy" to the rest of the world. We are told by our leaders that our way of life must be forced upon the rest of the world whether they like it or not because it is the right thing to do. I got news for you folks, you need to go study a little. Our country was NEVER intended to be a democracy. It was founded as a "Republic" form of government. And do you notice those two words? Democracy(Democrat) and Republic(Republican) and the similarities. Remember what I said about words, are they not very clever? The fact of the matter is we are no longer either one. We are an Oligarchy. Go look it up. You really need to do a little research on your own. It makes you more likely to retain it.

Most of you are not aware that when it comes to our government, there are now actually two of them. But that is a discussion for another day. The government and corporations seem to be devoid of any morality and spirituality. Yet they are the two greatest influences on this world we call earth. Governments rule and corporations produce and profit from all the commercial activity generated to meet our needs and desires. Both have been involved in the greatest down falls of mankind whether it be war or disease. The love of money and power are unsurpassed in the history of man. Again I say it is very simple, Satan using the tools of this earth to defeat us. There is certainly truth in the old saying "Money is Power". Just ask the Rothschilds, they will tell you. As N.M. Rothschild once said, "Let me but control a nation's currency, and I care not who makes it's laws". Our countries' National Debt is quickly approaching twenty trillion dollars and we all know all the ways that affects our lives. Yet the accumulated wealth of just one family, the Rothschilds is estimated to be approximately five hundred trillion dollars.

Look at all the law books and legal documents written and based in the Latin language. I guess no one ever told the justice system we speak English in this country. Just a carryover from the old days I imagine. It does not matter that you do not understand a damn thing without their interpretation and guidance. Could it be that the whole thing was created to keep you in the dark and ignorant of how the law works. It makes you dependent upon them to make the underpinnings of the legal system work. I am sure there have been good men who have made justice in law there life's goal. Men who had good intentions as they started their careers but did not last long in the study and practice of law because they would not play the game. I would even venture to say that some even found their life to be short lived if you know what I mean. I am not a Bible thumping scripture slinging man, but I do know there is a part of it devoted to the discussion of Judges. When it comes to you and your health, there is so much money involved that there is an endless line of people just waiting for their piece of the pie. It is enough to make you sick, no pun intended. The one that really gets me angry is when we start to use all this at the expense of the health of children.

There are organizations that have been a part of the whole "Charitable" thing and giving. With information about these institutions more easily accessed these days, we have found out that the largest portion of the money we were giving to these "age old" institutions was actually going to enrich the bank accounts of those running the damn things and the day to day operations which guaranteed their continued existence. These are people who were supposed to be those wonderful upstanding people who were "Devoting their Lives" to helping others. I will tell you that all this is only a small part of why health care costs so much. I am sure you have all heard of the four dollars you were charged for a single Aspirin at the hospital. And if the corporations and big Parma are not ripping us off, the regulations imposed on them and us by government are making up for anything they forgot. Our health is important to our continuation as a species. I am sure there are those who live in the ivory tower that just look at us common men as some kind of parasite. Leaching and living an existence that is depriving them of the things "THEY" feel they are entitled to as they feel they are a better class of people.

We are now at a point where corporations have the same rights as people. That is because our system of law in now based in Commercial Law and not the Common Law that was the basis for our Constitution. Corporations are not human beings. They cannot have the God given rights rooted in our spirituality and humanity that is us as a species. Rights given to us by God and not some men in a place called the Congress or United Nations. The fact of the matter is, that piece of paper even says so and it is STILL the highest form of law in the land contrary to what some may have you believe. I hope everyone is getting their money's worth from the "Representatives" we send to Washington D.C. again and again. Man's law had become a joke. It has become so manipulated and confusing that even the judges and lawyers cannot understand it, let alone the common man. Words have come to mean whatever some judicial person says they mean today. Remember those infamous words once said by one of our former Presidents, "That is according to what the meaning of the word is, is". Well he was right, that IS the way law works now. Words interpreted by men whose egos make them feel they are entitled to impose their will on everyone else by virtue of their position in the legal system. This is judicial activism hard at work.

But I digress with my rambling. We are supposed to be talking about Cancer here right? This is kind of my point. I do not pretend to know our last President. I have never met the man but I cannot help but feel he is a man driven by bitterness and misguided ideals doing exactly the opposite of what he says he is. A man who became President and rammed what is now one of the largest fiascos in history down our throats for the benefit of his own place in history. The Affordable Care Act. It was created in haste for the benefit of those thirty some odd million people at the expense of the other three hundred eighty million people who live in this country. Socialism at its best folks and you better get used to it because there is much more of this sort of thing to come. Look at the turmoil and division it has created in a country. It is destroying our medical system, people's health and their lives. As the Congress stands divided by party loyalty and the desire to be reelected, arguing like a bunch of spoiled children in the school yard fighting over a ball. I knew we were in trouble when this President's wife stood up in front of thousands and said that for the first time in her life she was proud to be an American after her husband was elected. In other words she was ashamed to be an American before but now that they were running the show, everything was great. And the worst part is that those thousands of idiots in the audience clapped and clapped for her. They have created a racial divide that is so large I do not know if we will ever be united as a country again.

God's law never changes. It is rooted in our spirits. It is unwavering, constant and dependable. It always has been and always will be. Well you have heard pretty much all that I have to say. I guess I will leave it at that for now. I think you get the picture as to how all this is affecting your health. Got a headache yet? I would say that if we do not all wake up and make some pretty big changes we are going to be up the proverbial creek without a paddle. Quite honestly, I am not sure that we are not past the point of no return now. That is why I have started to devote my life to finding that next plane of existence and doing what I need to do to get there so when I die, my spirit will move on to whatever that amazing place may be, Lord willing. As for your health and your battle with Cancer, hang in there folks, it ain't over yet!

CLOSING

I hope you were able to read this book and think about your battle with Cancer and how you can truly affect a change in your life spiritually, mentally and physically. I look at it from the viewpoint that even if a few lives are changed and extended I will have been a success. Hopefully maybe a few souls saved too. I want this book to be a help to you. I love you as my fellow man and want you to live as long and full a life as you possibly can. There is life after Cancer as I like to tell people. I am a walking testimony to that fact. I firmly believe you can achieve it if you just try as hard as you can and reach out to God and try to make the connection. At this point you have to ask yourself, "What have I got to lose?" At the very least enjoy the time you have left to the fullest and leave this life knowing that the world is a better place for your having been in it. I cannot stress enough that you must reach out to God and others with everything you have. For many of you, this will be no easy task, but you CAN do it!

Those of you who are capable, make a Bucket List. Do some of the things you have always wanted to do, within the capabilities of your current condition of course. DO NOT roll over and play dead. At the risk of sounding a bit melodramatic, cry out to God in heavens in search of his help and guidance. Do not let others dictate what you can and cannot do. When you have Cancer, many may try to manipulate you into doing what they want or some doctor says is best. Every situation is different and only YOU know what your limitations are right now. I say this in regards to the people around you. Some may be overprotective because they love you. Some may just do things because it makes THEIR life easier and the situation you have presented them with easier. You must approach this with tact and sensible discussion. They may feel you are not well enough to make your own decisions or have a different perspective than you do concerning your condition. If you exercise common sense and use science, strength and God's help to their fullest, I believe with all my heart you will either live longer or at least be at peace with what may be coming. Any way you look at it, you win. In any regard, wherever you are in your battle with Cancer, the time you have left will be the best it can possibly be and would be willing to bet that God will take notice. God bless you and be well my friends. LIVE ON!!!!!

I have added this at the very end. I have decided that if this book does actually get published and make any money, I am going to donate fifty percent of the first two years earnings to the St. Judes Children's Hospital for Cancer in Indianapolis, Indiana. Those children need all the help they can get! God love you.

Printed in the United States
By Bookmasters